CLINICAL NOTES IN VASCULITIC DISEASES

Dr. Faisael Albalwi
And
Dr. Ibrahim Alhomood
Dr. Fatemah Binladen
Pharmacist Fahad Albalawi

Order this book online at www.trafford.com
or email orders@trafford.com

Most Trafford titles are also available at major online book retailers.

© Copyright 2022 Dr. Faisael Albalwi.
All rights reserved. No part of this publication may be reproduced, stored in a retrieval system, or transmitted, in any form or by any means, electronic, mechanical, photocopying, recording, or otherwise, without the written prior permission of the author.

Print information available on the last page.

ISBN: 978-1-6987-1232-1 (sc)
ISBN: 978-1-6987-1234-5 (hc)
ISBN: 978-1-6987-1233-8 (e)

Library of Congress Control Number: 2022913426

Because of the dynamic nature of the Internet, any web addresses or links contained in this book may have changed since publication and may no longer be valid. The views expressed in this work are solely those of the author and do not necessarily reflect the views of the publisher, and the publisher hereby disclaims any responsibility for them.

Any people depicted in stock imagery provided by Getty Images are models, and such images are being used for illustrative purposes only.
Certain stock imagery © Getty Images.

Trafford rev. 11/12/2022

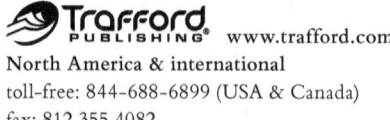 www.trafford.com

North America & international
toll-free: 844-688-6899 (USA & Canada)
fax: 812 355 4082

CONTENTS

Dedication vii

Preface ix

(1) The First Chapter 1
Systemic Approach to The Patients with
Suspected Vasculitic Diseases:

(2) The Second Chapter 7
An Overview of Vasculitic Diseases:

(3) The Third Chapter 147
Therapeutic Agents in Management of Vasculitis

(4) The Fourth Chapter 160
Test Yourself (Short Real Cases)

References 163

DEDICATION

To my parents, the greatest teachers in the world
To my wife and my son Turki, the light of my life
To all Rheumatologists who have the interest in Vasculitis

PREFACE

This is a simplified book that concentrates on different vasculitic diseases seen in the clinical practice. Hopefully, the book will guide rheumatology trainees for better understanding of vasculitis.

(1) THE FIRST CHAPTER

SYSTEMIC APPROACH TO THE PATIENTS WITH SUSPECTED VASCULITIC DISEASES:

★★Systemic Vasculitic Disorders:

★Introduction:

- Vasculitis: systemic inflammatory process affecting the walls of blood vessels and causing wide spectrum of systemic manifestations.
- The manifestations of these vasculitic inflammatory disorders arise from one or both of the following mechanisms:

(A) When the inflammation occurs due to inflammatory cells infiltrate, walls of blood vessels will be thinner and easy to rupture: Small-Vessel Vasculitis; *or*

(B) As a result of severe inflammatory reaction with intimal proliferation, narrowing and occlusion of the blood vessels will appear and ischemic symptoms will happen: Large or Medium-Vessel Vasculitis.

★*Points should be considered when you are thinking about vasculitic diseases in ill patients:*

1– *Is it a primary vasculitic disorder or a mimicker condition?*
2– *If it is a primary vasculitis, what is the most likely subtype?*
3– *What is the extent of this vasculitic disease?*
4– *What are the tests that should be requested to confirm the diagnosis?*

**Names for vasculitides adopted by the 2012 International Chapel Hill Consensus Conference on the Nomenclature of Vasculitides:

===

Large vessel vasculitis (LVV)
Takayasu arteritis (TAK)
Giant cell arteritis (GCA)

Medium vessel vasculitis (MVV)
Polyarteritis nodosa (PAN)
Kawasaki disease (KD)

Small vessel vasculitis (SVV)
<u>Antineutrophil cytoplasmic antibody ANCA–associated vasculitis (AAV):</u>
Microscopic polyangiitis (MPA)
Granulomatosis with polyangiitis (Wegener's) (GPA)
Eosinophilic granulomatosis with polyangiitis (Churg-Strauss) (EGPA)

<u>Immune complex SVV:</u>
Anti–glomerular basement membrane (anti-GBM) disease
Cryoglobulinemic vasculitis (CV)
IgA vasculitis (Henoch-Schonlein Purpura) (IgAV)
Hypocomplementemic urticarial vasculitis (HUV) (anti-C1q vasculitis)

Variable vessel vasculitis (VVV)
Behcet's disease (BD)
Cogan's syndrome (CS)

Single-organ vasculitis (SOV)
Cutaneous leukocytoclastic angiitis
Cutaneous arteritis
Primary central nervous system vasculitis
Isolated aortitis
Others

Vasculitis associated with systemic disease
Lupus vasculitis
Rheumatoid vasculitis
Sarcoid vasculitis
Others

Vasculitis associated with probable etiology
Hepatitis C virus–associated cryoglobulinemic vasculitis
Hepatitis B virus–associated vasculitis
Syphilis-associated aortitis
Drug-associated immune complex vasculitis
Drug-associated ANCA-associated vasculitis
Cancer-associated vasculitis
Others

DR. FAISAEL ALBALWI

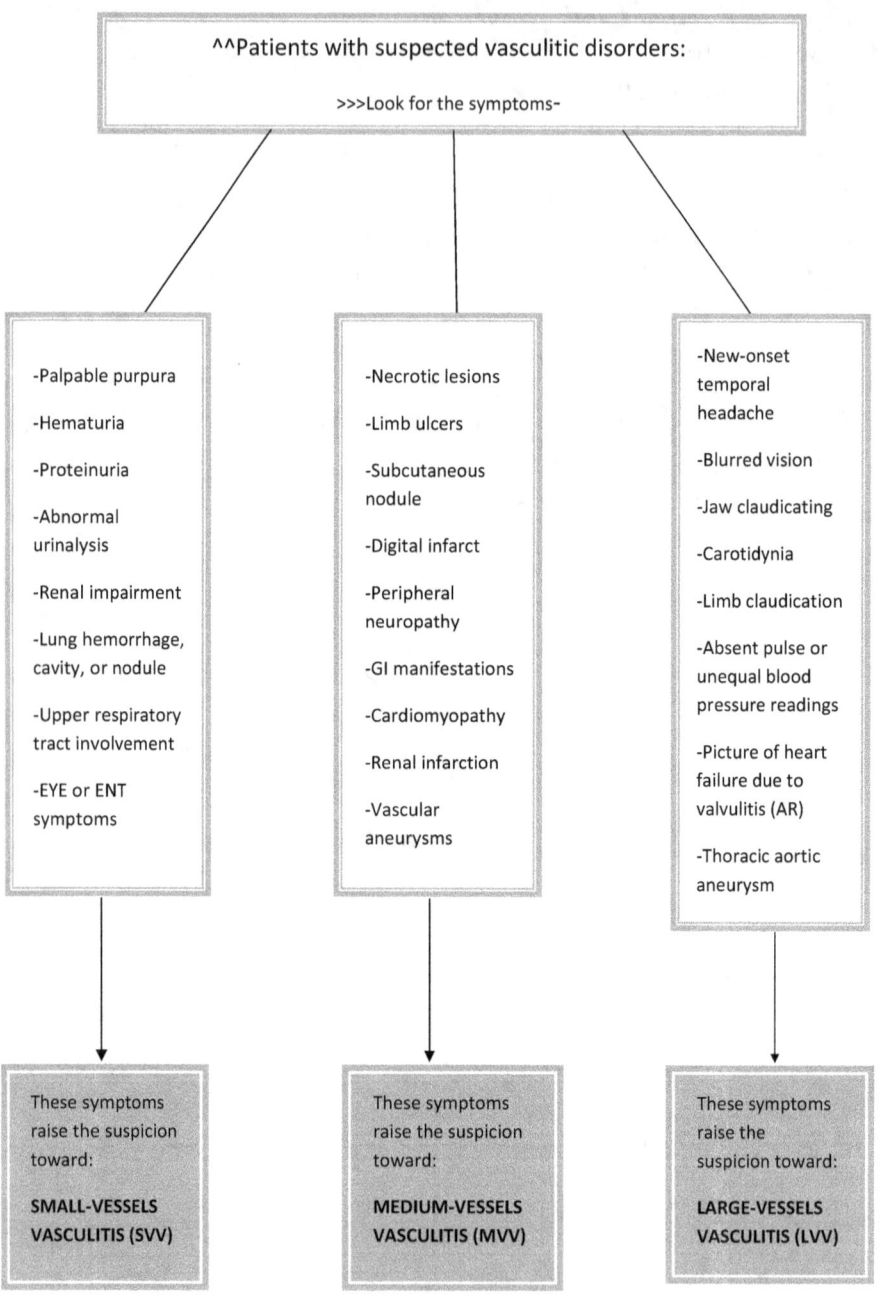

CLINICAL NOTES IN VASCULITIC DISEASES

★Investigations should be ordered when you are seeing the patients suspected to have a primary vasculitic disorder:-

1– CBC with differentials: Leukocytosis or high platelets are seen among patients with active disease. Moreover, anemia of chronic disease might be noticed.
2– Renal and Hepatic profiles: to check if there is rise in serum creatinine or increment in hepatic enzymes.
3– Urinalysis and urine toxicology: to detect any abnormal urine sediment, and also twenty-four-hour urine protein collection is important.
4– ESR/CRP: These are not specific markers. However, they may rise during active disease.
5– Full septic screen: Extremely important to be done to avoid infectious process.
6– Hepatitis B or Hepatitis C serology: As they are associated with development of specific subtypes of vasculitic diseases.
7– HIV or varicella serology: May cause a clinical condition-like vasculitis (CNS vasculitis).
8– COVID-19 PCR: This is a newer viral agent that can cause different systemic condition including vasculitis mimickers.
9– Serology for syphilis: VDRL or TPHA. Patients with *syphilitic disease* can present with vasculitis (especially aortitis).
10– QuantiFERON-TB: It is considered an important infectious agent that can manifest with a picture of vasculitis-like phenomenon.
11– Autoimmune work-up should be done: ANA, complements, ANCA, and cryoglobulins.
12– Chest X-ray (CXR) and high-resolution CT-Chest (HRCT-chest): To recognize any lung lesions (infiltrate, nodules, cavity?).
13– Transthoracic echocardiogram: For assessment cardiac function and to rule out vasculitis mimicker like infective endocarditis.

*Confirmatory tests used to manage primary vasculitic disorders:

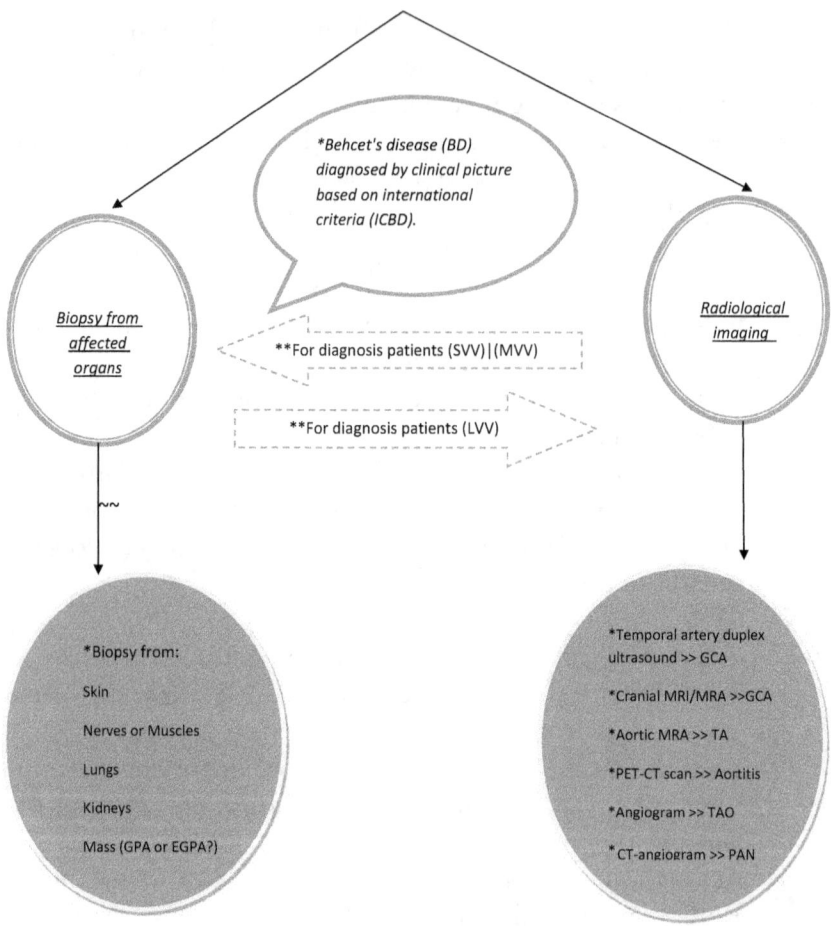

(2) THE SECOND CHAPTER

AN OVERVIEW OF VASCULITIC DISEASES:

^^Large Vessels Vasculitis

Giant Cell Arteritis

★Introduction:

A- GCA is the most prevalent systemic vasculitis in adults.
B- It is a disease commonly found in older age group above fifty years (mostly seen in their sixties to seventies).
C- More in females 2–4:1.
D- Obviously, it involves extracranial branches of carotid artery and it can involves the aorta + major branches.
E- However, Intracranial vasculitis reported in the literature

★Pathogenesis:

A- It is a granulomatous inflammation that depends on (Th1 and Th17) in its occurrence.
B- The initiating stimulant could be either: genetic defect (HLA-DRB1★04) or infectious agent (Mycoplasma pneumonia or Varicella-Zoster).
C- After that, the dendritic cells and macrophages in innate immune system will be activated and they will release (IL-12 and IL-23 to stimulate Th1) and (IL-1B and IL-6 to stimulate Th17).

D- As a result of that, Th1 cells will release >>> IFN-G and TNF-A, stimulating vascular smooth muscle cells.
E- Also, Th17 cells will release IL-17, IL-21, IL-22, or IL-23 that helps in collaboration with Th1 cytokines:

^ inflammatory cells infiltrate with production of matrix metalloproteinase enzymes >>> leads to damage of tunica media and internal elastic lamina,
^ vascular smooth muscle cells proliferation >>> leads to occlusion (Ischemia),
^ stimulate hepatocytes for production of acute phase reactants, and
^ VDGF-stimulation for neoangiogenesis >>> to help in reducing the symptoms of ischemia.

*Clinical Assessment:

– By history:

1– new onset (severe) headache\scalp pain which is located in the temporal or occipital areas (70 percent),
2– symptoms of stroke,
3– jaw, tongue claudication, or dysphagia,
4– visual symptoms like amaurosis fugax, considered the highest predictive factor for permanent vision loss (also diplopia and ptosis have been reported),
5– limbs claudication and easy fatiguability upon limb movement with involvement of aorta and its major branches (15–20 percent and could be silent!),
6– chest pain and upper back pain,
7– constitutional symptoms: weight loss, low-grade fever, chronic cough, and don't forget to ask about any chronic comorbidities (DM, HTN),
8– don't forget to ask about PMR symptoms (like hip or shoulder girdles stiffness), and
9– any points suggestive for malignancy.

– By Examination:

1– Examine for temporal areas tenderness, cordlike temporal artery, and reduced temporal artery pulses.
2– Look for scalp necrosis and assess for shoulder or hip girdles stiffness *(not weakness)*.
3– Look for any difference in pulse or BP or vascular bruits.
4– Important to do: fundoscopy, or better to call an ophthalmologist to assess for retinal ischemia or papilledema (AION-arteritic).
5– Any signs for malignancy >>> lymph nodes enlargement.

*ACR 1990 diagnostic criteria for GCA (More than or equal to three) (Sen. 93.5 percent and Spe. 91.2 percent):

- age more than or equal to fifty years,
- new onset headache,
- temporal artery tenderness or decreased in pulsation,
- ESR more than or equal 50, and/or
- positive temporal artery biopsy.

*Investigations:

Basic laboratory:

1– CBC+diff. >>> Anemia of chronic disease or high platelets >>> positive phase reactant,
2– Renal profile and urine analysis >>> Any proteinuria! *(Why?)*,
3– Hepatic profile: transaminitis or high ALP (mild) >>> should improve with treatment,
4– ESR: more than or equal 50 mm/hr in 88 percent or 10 percent of the patients with ESR < 50 *(only 2–3 percent will have normal ESR!)*,
5– CRP is elevated in majority of the patients,
6– SPEP/UPEP rule out plasma cell dyscrasias, and
7– Hep. B, hep. C, HIV, or QuantiFERON-TB to be requested.

Basic Imaging (within one week after starting steroid)

1- Temporal artery duplex ultrasound +\- axillary artery >>> (non-compressible halo sign >>> Sen. 75 percent and Sp.83 percent),
2- High resolution cranial MRI can be used for diagnosis if ultrasound is not available, and to determine any narrowed segments in cranial arteries,
3- MRA-aorta, CTA, or PET-CT >>> used to detect aortitis in the aorta and its major branches' involvement, and
4- transthoracic echo is important to know if there is any aortic valve dilation >>> (AR).

Pathological assessment *(gold standard test)*:

★★Temporal artery biopsy (within one week after starting steroid) is better to be done bilaterally, to be taken with a long segment of 3 cm–5 cm as it's a patchy disease to improve diagnostic accuracy (Sen=85–88 percent), and negative biopsy doesn't exclude the disease if GCA is highly suspected.

★★Finding in biopsy: 50 percent granulomatous inflammation with multinucleated giant cells. Other finding: mononuclear cells infiltrate or mixed infiltrate (lymphocytes and macrophages) >>> *fibrinoid necrosis and neutrophils are not seen in biopsy of patients with GCA.*

★★Don't do temporal artery biopsy if the patient presented is with aortitis and doesn't have any headache or jaw claudication, as > 40 percent of the patients will have negative biopsy (image: MRA, CTA, or PET-CT are good!).

Simplified approach for diagnosis of (GCA):

High clinical suspicion of (GCA with typical headache and typical jaw claudication, etc. and very high inflammatory markers).

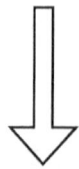

Request temporal artery duplex (expert operator) >>> If positive, no need for biopsy and treat GCA. But if US is negative and the patient is highly suspected,

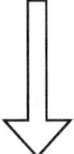

You can request high-resolution head and neck cranial MRI. If positive, treat the patient as GCA.

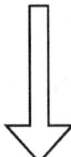

If both imaging modalities were negative or not available and the patient is highly suspected, *go for biopsy!*

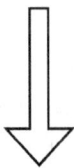

If the patient is considered low risk as (headache on and off and ESR is not rising significantly), do any imaging modalities (temporal artery duplex or cranial MRI) If negative image, don't proceed and look for another differential.

★★Differential diagnoses in a case with GCA:

1– Chronic infections such as TB, HIV, subacute bacterial endocarditis.
2– RA: ask about symptoms of synovitis.
3– Malignancies: hematological (MM) or solid.
4– PMR: *ask about stiffness disturbing the life of the patient!*

5– NAAION: non-arteritic phenomenon which is seen commonly among individuals with age above fifty years and happened due to hypoperfusion in posterior ciliary branches. Risk factors: DM, HTN, high cholesterol, OSA, hypercoagulable state, and medications such as PDE-5 inhibitors.

6– *Amyloidosis* >>> *urianaysis* or immunoelectrophoresis: amyloid can cause jaw claudication occasionally.

*Management of GCA *(steroid* is first *line,* and once you are suspecting GCA, start steroid immediately):

A- Is there any vision threatening symptoms (amaurosis fugax, diplopia, or blurred vision)? If *yes,*

>>Therapy should be started by giving the patient pulse steroid therapy (IV methylprednisolone 15 mg/kg daily for three days), then 1 mg/kg oral prednisolone up to 60 mg PO OD and add steroid sparing agent.

B- If there is no vision threatening symptoms, the patients can be divided into two groups:

- First group: No history of any comorbidities—start prednisolone orally 1 mg/kg as monotherapy, then taper steroid therapy gradually.
- Second group: Positive history of comorbidities like DM, HTN, Second group: Positive history of comorbidities like DM, HTN, osteoporosis or other organs involvement such as: AORTITIS—start prednisolone orally 1 mg/kg and steroid sparing agent.

C- Regarding steroid therapy, start to decrease the dose gradually after one month when the symptoms improve and inflammatory markers decline to reach 20 mg at three months, then to reach 5 mg PO OD at one year.

D- In case of inability to taper steroid or relapsing disease or positive history for comorbidities, use steroid sparing agent.

E- Regarding steroid sparing agents:

- First line: tocilizumab (162 mg) SC once weekly. Fifty-six percent of the patients have sustained remission at fifty-two weeks, with reduction in both relapse rate 23 percent and in cumulative steroid dose as It had been shown in (GIACTA) trial.
- Methotrexate can be used based on meta-analysis that showed MTX can decrease the risk of relapse and reduce steroid dose.
- In case of relapse although previously mentioned meds have been started:

Abatacept can be used based on study from US showed relapse, free remission at fifty-two weeks up to 48 percent compared to steroid alone.

Ustekinumab is another option, and its use has been taken from small sized open-label study that showed no relapse, decrease steroid dose, and radiological improvement in large vessels vasculitis.

*JAKi >>> undergoing trials, like tofacitinib or baricitinib.

F- Aspirin therapy among all patients with GCA is advised, especially in case of vision threatening symptoms, or the patients carry a risk of cardiovascular or cerebrovascular diseases. It can be initiated after outweighing risks and benefits.

G- Educate the patient about the disease and explain that this disease will take a longer time for follow-up.

H- Vaccination and osteoporosis prophylaxis *(Important!)*.

#MONITORING the patients with GCA:

1- Follow the patient every one to three months initially, then every three to six months in case of stable disease. *Ask about ischemia symptoms and inflammatory markers* (the risk of relapse is about 50 percent).
2- Ask about steroid side effects, like DM, HTN, or osteoporosis (DEXA scan to be done).

3– Stabilize DM, HTN, dyslipidemia as patients with GCA have a high risk for atherosclerotic vascular disease.
4– Do MRA of the aorta and its major branches at the time of GCA diagnosis, then every two years to be sure that patients don't have any aortic inflammation or aneurysm, as patients with GCA have seventeen times higher risk for thoracic aortic aneurysm and two times higher risk for AAA. However, in case of high risk of aortic aneurysm, such as HTN, dyslipidemia, PMR symptoms, high ESR>100, or aortic regurgitation, do MRA every six months +\- echo.
5– In case patients with GCA have atypical symptoms or refractoriness to steroid therapy, which is uncommon in GCA patients, request ANCA profile and look for fibrinoid necrosis in biopsy. *False pure GCA?*

==

Takayasu's Arteritis (TA):

*Introduction:

A- Chronic granulomatous vascular inflammation that affects large vessels, mainly aorta and its major branches.

B- It affects young-aged patients (more than 90 percent females) with age twenty to forty years.

C- It causes luminal narrowing with picture of ischemia and aneurismal formation.

*Pathogenesis:

A- The occurrence of TA is dependent on cell mediated immunity with mainly T-helper cells and NKT cells.

B- Genetic predisposition may play a role HLA-B39\HLA-B52.

C- Recently proven that even B lymphocytes participate in injury of blood vessels (anti-endothelial cell antibodies).

D- The inflammation happened mainly in the tunica adventitia and tunica media with persistent inflammation leads to stenosis of blood vessels

*Clinical Assessment :-

By history:

    1– hypertension *(renovascular)*,
    2– limb claudication,
    3– TIA or stroke: involvement of carotid or vertebral arteries,
    4– constitutional symptoms like fatigue, weight loss, and fever,
    5– dizziness during exertion due to reduced cerebral blood flow,
    6– chest pain as a result of coronary artery involvement,

7– myoarthralgia is noticed among patients with TA, and *don't forget to ask about symptoms of SPA*. Spondyloarthropathies can cause aortitis!
8– history about diabetes, dyslipidemia, and smoking,
9– neck pain upon touching the skin,
10– cough or hemoptysis rarely happened due to pulmonary arteritis (uncommon)!
11– abdominal pain and diarrhea >>> mesenteric ischemia (uncommon),
12– any history of drug abuse. *Cocaine induces vascular spasm!*
13– erythema nodosum is reported among minority of patients with TA.

By Exam:

1– Difference in pulse.
2– Difference in BP with >10 mm Hg between two arms.
3– Carotidynia with allodynia while touching the patient's neck.
4– Any murmur, look for aortic regurgitation!
5– Listen for any bruits.
6– Any rash or evidence of synovitis. Also, back examination is important!
7– Any features of Marfan syndrome or hypermobility of the joints, EDS.
8– Any lymphadenopathy >>> R/O (TB).

**ACR 1990 classification criteria for Takayasu's Arteritis (TA): (Se. 90 percent & Spe. 97percent) (more than or equal to three, suggestive for TA)

1– Age at onset of disease less than or equal to forty years.
2– Claudication of the extremities: worsening of pain or fatigue during use.
3– Decreased pulse in the brachial artery.
4– Systolic BP difference >10 mm Hg between two arms.
5– Presence of bruits in the subclavian artery or abdominal aorta.
6– Angiograpgic abnormality: stenosis or occlusion of aorta (focal or segmental).

CLINICAL NOTES IN VASCULITIC DISEASES

*Investigations:

Basic Labs:

1– CBC: Chronic anemia, high platelets count;
2– Renal and hepatic profiles: High creatinine could be related HTN from renal artery involvement;
3– ESR is a useful marker in context of vasculitis, but can be normal in active disease;
4– CRP can rise during active process;
5– HbA1c, lipid profile >>> atherosclerosis?
6– Hepatitis B and C serology;
7– HIV, QuantiFERON-TB, and syphilis testing;
8– Urine screening for illicit drug abuse.

Basic Imaging:

1– *Angiography* is the gold standard image for diagnosis; however, not any more recommended as it's an invasive procedure and has been replaced by other modalities. It can detect narrowing or occlusion or aneurysm.
2– *Magnetic Resonance Angiography:* the modality of choice as recommended by (EULAR), and the advantages include:

^ ability to detect early vascular inflammation, such as wall edema or thickening, and
^ Can detect narrowing or stenosis or aneurysms.

3– *Computed Tomography Angiography*: another modality can be utilized for diagnosing TA, as it can give us an idea about the lumen and blood flow inside the vasculature.
4– *Transthoracic echo:* advised to be requested to determine any aortic regurgitation or assessment of cardiac function.

*Pathological assessment:

It is not necessary to be done as clinical feature, and imaging is considered enough for diagnosis. However the biopsy of inflamed blood vessel revealed:

- ^ thickening of adventitia,
- ^ leukocytes inflammation in tunica media and adventitia, and
- ^ intimal hyperplasia.

★Simplified approach for diagnosis (TA):

If a young patient is complaining of (HTN) or symptoms of claudication or any feature of ischemia,

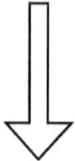

Take full history and try to exclude other differentials, then do full examination.

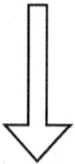

Request basic labs and imaging. MRA is recommended due to its ability to detect inflammation and for less radiation exposure.

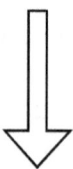

If other differentials have been excluded and MRA image has shown picture of inflammation, consider *Takayasu's Disease*.

★Differential diagnosis in case with TA:

1– Atherosclerosis >>> Ask for history of diabetes, smoking, and cardiovascular disease.

CLINICAL NOTES IN VASCULITIC DISEASES

2– Ehler-Danlos syndrome or Marfan syndrome >>> Look for joint hypermobility, marfanoid habitus, and abnormal scarring. Genetic testing is important.

3– Fibromuscular dysplasia >>> The patient will have high BP with reduced pulse. However, angiogram will show beading appearance of the affected vessels.

4– Infections such as *syphilis* >>> Do serological testing, and CTA will show calcification in the aorta. *Tuberculosis is another possibility.*

5– Spondyloarthropathies can cause aortic inflammation.

★Management of TA:

A- The aim in Takayasu's arteritis is to suppress inflammation, improve systemic symptoms, and prevent further damage.

B- Treatment consists of higher dose of steroid (1 mg/kg) 60 mg PO OD and additional immunosuppressive medication since beginning, as the disease carries a high risk of relapse. For tapering, it should be done after one month and to reach 20 mg/day by twelve weeks, with the dose to be less than or equal to 10 mg PO once a day at twelve months.

C- Examples of immunosuppressive medications that can be used:

- Methotrexate (MTX = 15 mg weekly): The use of MTX based on different case series which revealed a good clinical response and retarding of radiographic progression.
- Azathioprine (2 mg/kg): Azathioprine is proven to improve clinical response and normalize inflammatory markers with stability of radiographic finding.
- Mycophenolate Mofetil (MMF 1.5 to 2 g/day): MMF is considered a good option as steroid sparing agent with an acceptable safety profile as has been studied in Chinese cohort that involved thirty patients with clinical resolution and radiographic progression has been retarded.
- *CYCLOPHOSPHAMIDE* can be used in case of refractoriness.

D- In case of relapse or refractory disease, consider using TNF-inhibitors as per case series, which showed clinical improvement with normalization of inflammatory markers and retardation of radiographic progression.

E- Regarding tocilizumab, it is not a suitable choice as in case of GCA, but there are some studies that showed some improvement in clinical symptoms and inflammatory markers.

F- Interestingly, *rituximab* (RTX) is used to treat some Takayasu's arteritis patients with refractory pattern, as per some case reports.

G- Tofacitinib is considered a promising agent for treating patients with refractory disease (TA) based on recent data.

H- *Vascular intervention,* either by endovascular intervention or open surgical reconstruction, is needed when the patient has:

#hypertension with difficulty to control,
#enlarging vascular aneurysms,
#aortic regurgitation.

Consultation with vascular surgeons should be arranged, and better to arrange surgery during remission of disease.

I- Vaccination and osteoporosis prophylaxis.

I- Aspirin generally should not be given to all patients unless there is high risk for cardiovascular disease like IHD or stroke.

*Monitoring of patients with TA:

1– It is advised to do close follow-up during active disease every one to three months. Then if the disease is stable, every three to six months.
2– The need for follow-up by image (MRA, CTA, or ultrasound duplex) is guided by doing watchful approach for occlusion or aneurysm every now and then from six to twelve months.

3– Ask about symptoms of ischemia, like Claudication, stroke, angina symptoms, ESR/CRP, and systemic symptoms.
4– Don't forget to ask about sequelae of TA, such as aortic regurgitation symptoms, cardiac ischemia, pulmonary hypertension, pulmonary thrombosis, cerebral ischemia, renal artery stenosis with persistent uncontrolled HTN, and retinal ischemia.
5– Don't depend on ESR/CRP for diagnosis of relapse, as they can be normal during active disease.
6– In case of persistent elevation in inflammatory markers, the approach to rule out: infection with extensive workup, and if the workup came back negative, do imaging.
7– The prognosis in TA: the patients carry a high risk for relapse of more than 50 percent. In relation to survival rate, this is based on Japanese cohort of 120 patients, with fifteen years survival rate reaching up to 82.9 percent.

★Takayasu's Disease and Pregnancy:

^ Pregnancy will not cause an aggressive attack of vasculitis.
^ The most important thing is that the pregnancy should occur during remission phase with pregnancy compatible medications.
^ Check the cardiac and renal functions, and management of HTN should be optimal to avoid maternal complications of hypertension, such as preeclampsia.
^ Check for aortic regurgitation and aortic aneurysms before pregnancy.
^ There is an increased risk of fetal loss by 15 percent, with risk of preterm birth.
^ Multidisciplinary teams' approach is paramount (rheumatologist, obstetrician, vascular surgeon, and cardiologist).

===

*Aortitis: *classified under single organ vasculitis*

*Introduction:

A- Aortitis: a term that involves all conditions that can cause inflammation of the aorta.

B- The prevalence of aortitis varies, and based on one retrospective study which collected (1204) specimens from the aorta post-surgical intervention, either due to aneurismal dilation or dissection, they found the following:

- 4.3 percent = fifty-two cases of the patients have idiopathic aortitis,
- 67 percent of the patients were women with mean age of sixty-three years, and
- 31 percent = sixteen cases of patients with idiopathic aortitis have prior history of systemic illness, while 69 percent of the patients don't have any systemic disease.

C- The classification of aortitis is dependent on the burden of inflammation:

#Type I: inflammation in the aortic arch and its branches.
#Type IIa: inflammation includes ascending aorta, aortic arch, and its branches.
#Type IIb: same extent as in type IIa and descending thoracic aorta.
#Type III: involvement of descending thoracic aorta, abdominal aorta, and renal arteries.
#Type IV: involvement of abdominal aorta and renal arteries.
#Type V: features of type IIb and type IV.

D- The major subtypes of aortitis: Infectious Vs. Noninfectious

Pathogenesis:

1- In the same manner as in cases of GCA/TA, there is inflammatory T-cell infiltrate with different subtypes.
2- This infiltration will cause different complications, such as vascular occlusion or intimal fibrosis, causing ischemic symptoms.

3– The condition in case of infectious aortitis is different and focusing on infection of atheromatous plaques, or embolization from nidus of infection (IE), or contagious spread of overwhelming infection, or bacterial contamination post vascular surgery or trauma.

*Etiology:

>>Non-Infectious aortitis:

1– Large vessels vasculitis (GCA/TA) are the most common causes of non-infectious aortitis. (Be careful that even PMR alone can be associated with aortitis!)
2– Variable vessels vasculitis like Behcet's disease or Cogan's syndrome.
3– Relapsing polychondritis, rheumatoid arthritis, SLE, or HLA-B27 associated SpA.
4– Sarcoidosis based on case reports.
5– Chronic periaortitis (retropertoneal fibrosis or Inflammatory abdominal aortic aneurysm).
6– IgG4-related disease can present with aortic inflammation.
7– Radiation exposure.
8– Medications like methysergide, bevacizumab combination chemotherapy protocol.
9– Idiopathic phenotype: more related to female gender, history of heavy smoking, and family history of aortic aneurysm.

>>Infectious aortitis: Ask about any history of DM, cancer, immunosuppressive drugs, alcoholism, IV drugs abuse, sexual history, travel history, and raw milk ingestion.

1– Gram-positive cocci >>> staphylococci, streptococcus pneumoniae, or enterococcus;
2– Salmonella;
3– Mycobacterium TB;
4– Treponema pallidum >>> syphilis;
5– Brucella melitensis;
6– Listeria monocytogenes;
7– Nocardia asteroids;
8– Fungal organisms such as Candida and Aspergillus; and

9– Viral infections such as Hepatitis B and C, and HIV.

★Clinical assessment:

>Symptoms of GCA, TA, and Behcet's disease,
>Fever,
>Any ocular symptoms,
>Chest, back, or abdominal pain,
>Weight loss, and
>Symptoms of heart failure (due to aortic regurgitation).

★Investigations:

>>Basic labs:

1– CBC: to check for leukocytosis for infectious aortitis.
2– Renal profile and bone profile: check for hypercalcemia to rule out granulomatous disease.
3– Hepatic profile.
4– Blood culture: two sets of blood culture taken from two different places with difference in time of about one hour.
5– Acute phase reactants (ESR/CRP) will be elevated in majority of the patients.
6– Viral hepatitis serology.
7– HIV and syphilis serology.
8– ANA, anti-ds DNA, or complements.
9– Immunoglobulins level (IgG4 level), especially if the patient has periaortic fibrosis after ruling out lymphoma.
10– HLA-typing.

>>Basic imaging:

1– Computed tomography angiography (CTA): used to identify aortic wall abnormalities and can detect complications like aneurysm or aortic calcification.
2– Magnetic resonance angiography (MRA): useful in detection of early inflammation with better assessment for cardiac tissues.

3– Positron emission tomography (PET-CT): can detect active aortitis, and can be used for looking for extravascular nidus of infection.
4– Vascular duplex ultrasound (US): can be used to recognize some vascular inflammation in the temporal (halo sign), carotid, subclavian, and axillary arteries. Takayasu's disease can present with extensive wall thickening with brighter segment in comparison with halo sign.
5– Transthoracic echocardiography (TTE/TEE): to rule out vegetations, aortic regurgitation, aortic wall aneurysm, and abscess.

*Pathological assessment: (aortic segment taken during surgery) various histopathological findings are found:

- Granulomatous subtype: with marked macrophages involvement like GCA, TA, TB, and fungal infections.
- Lymphoplasmacytic subtype: lymphocytic infiltrate, mainly this pattern is seen in diseases like-IgG4-related disease, lupus, SpA, and Syphilis.
- Mixed inflammatory subtype: different inflammatory cells seen like Behcet's disease and Cogan's syndrome.
- Purulent subtype: dense neutrophilic infiltrate with presence of necrosis, and this phenomenon is seen in diseases like infectious aortitis.

*Simplified approach for diagnosis (Aortitis):

- If the patient has symptoms suggestive of aortitis like chest or back pain or discovered incidentally,
- Ask about symptoms of large vessels vasculitis, and other symptoms present in disorders like Behcet's disease, Cogan's syndrome, lupus, and infections like TB, syphilis, or persistent fever.
- Do basic labs and imaging mention before, especially blood cultures, (CTA/MRA), and echo.
- We are trying to identify what is the reason that could be a trigger for aortitis. If all differentials have been excluded, the disease is likely idiopathic in nature *(idiopathic isolated aortitis!)*.

*Management of Aortitis:

1– Once aortitis been diagnosed, therapy should be started as soon as possible to catch the patient earlier and to prevent development of complications, like aortic rupture.
2– Multidisciplinary approach is important: rheumatologist, cardiologist, ID doctor, and vascular surgeon.
3– In case of aortitis related to large vessels vasculitis, high dose steroid (1 mg/kg/day) tapered over months, +\- additional immunosuppressive medications with referral to surgery.
4– In case of infectious aortitis, IV antibiotics should be started immediately as this condition carries a high risk of mortality, even with treatment to cover both (staphylococci and gram-negative rods) for at least two to four weeks prior to surgery, then vascular intervention will be suitable, followed by six to twelve weeks of antimicrobial therapies dependent on culture post-surgery from the last negative culture. However, in case of persistent immunosuppressive status or some organisms, persistent antibiotic therapy can be used for long term.
5– Regarding idiopathic isolated aortitis, steroid course is important and surgical intervention.
6– Other diseases associated with aortitis to be treated as we are treating primary disease with high dose steroid and additional immunosuppressive therapies.
7– Vascular intervention (open vs. endovascular) to be decided by vascular surgery team, and advice to be arranged during inactive disease if the patient can wait.

*Monitoring for the patients with Aortitis: the visit to be scheduled every one to three months during active condition, then every three to six months.

^ Ask about symptoms like chest, abdominal, or back pain;
^ constitutional symptoms like fever;
^ ischemia symptoms like claudication, etc.;
^ follow inflammatory markers (to be done post-surgical intervention for long-term follow-up);
^ imaging like MRA every six to twelve months to look for appearance of new aneurismal dilation in other vascular territories.

^^Medium-Vessel Vasculitis:

*Polyarteritis Nodosa (PAN):

★Introduction:

- PAN is defined as segmental, transmural necrotizing arteritis affecting medium-sized blood vessels and sparing small arterioles and venules.
- Aneurysmal formation, ischemia, and limbs ulceration are sequelae that can happen among patients with PAN.
- PAN is seen commonly in middle-aged and older patients with ages in their forties to sixties.

★Pathogenesis:

- The pathophysiological mechanism behind occurrence of PAN is complex (most of primary cases of PAN are idiopathic).
- There are many environmental triggers that can induce the disease, like hepatitis B, parvo B19, Klebsiella, group a streptococci, toxoplasma, and HIV. Also, there are many other conditions being linked with development of PAN, such as hairy cell leukemia, RA, and Sjogren's syndrome.
- Those environmental antigens can enhance formation of immune-complex deposition, and this complex can turn on vascular inflammation with intimal proliferation, leading to ischemia, and softening of wall leading to aneurysm.
- Additionally, the impairment in regulation of immune system can induce production of different cytokines like TNF-a and IL-1b, with increased T-cell activity, causing systemic symptoms like malaise, weight loss, etc.
- Genetically, the defect (loss of function mutation) in the gene (CECR1) with deficiency in ADA2 enzyme can manifest with childhood PAN.

★Clinical Assessment:

- By History:

1– Ask about constitutional symptoms like fever, malaise, arthralgia, and weight loss.
2– New-onset HTN.
3– Risk factors for hepatitis B: drug abuse, blood transfusion, sexual contact.
4– Paraesthesia and weakness due to neuropathy (wrist or foot drop).
5– Picture of stroke (hemiplegia).
6– History of sudden loss of vision (come and go flashes!).
7– History of chest pain, shortness of breath: CHF secondary to coronary artery involvement.
8– History of abdominal pain, GI bleeding: be careful to identify acute abdomen early!
9– History of testicular swelling and pain (orchitis).
10– Cutaneous lesions: nodular erythematous lesion, ulcerative lesion, digital infarction, and livedo reticularis.

– By Examination:

1– Check the vitals: temperature and BP.
2– Cardiovascular examination.
3– Abdominal examination to R/O acute abdomen?
4– Neurological examination including fundoscopy. *Better to ask the help from ophthalmology.*
5– Check genitalia.
6– Check for cutaneous lesions.

*1990 ACR classification criteria for diagnosis (PAN) >>(Se=82 percent and Sp=86 percent) with three or more criteria:

1– Weight loss (non-intentional) more than or equal to 4 kg;
2– livedo reticularis;
3– testicular pain or tenderness;
4– positive hepatitis B serology;
5– myalgia mainly in the legs, leg tenderness;
6– mononeuropathy or polyneuropathy;
7– diastolic BP > 90 mm Hg;
8– rise in urea > 40 mg/dl and creatinine > 1.5 mg/dl;
9– angiographic abnormality showing aneurysm or occlusion;
10– biopsy showed medium vessels infiltration with neutrophils.

*Investigations:

>>>Basic labs:

1– CBC with differential >>> anemia of chronic disease or high platelets;
2– blood smear and SPEP >>> R/O hematological malignancies;
3– renal function test: check urea and creatinine;
4– urinalysis: proteinuria and hematuria due to renal ischemia and infarction *(no active urine sediment)*;
5– hepatic functions test: check for albumin and rise in LFT;
6– CPK level for myalgia;
7– inflammtory markers (ESR/CRP are high);
8– hepatitis B, hepatitis C, and HIV serologies;
9– blood cultures and QuantiFERON-TB testing;
10– ANCA testing should be *negative;*
11– cryoglobulin and complements level (patients with PAN can present with low complements);
12– electromyography and nerve conduction study: to recognize neuromyositis (mononeuritis multiplex is common among patients with PAN).

>>>Basic Imaging:

1– Visceral angiography: gold standard to detect microaneurysm in visceral circulation.
2– MRA/CTA: can be used in case of contraindication to invasive angiogram but can miss small aneurysms.
3– Echocardiogram (TTE): rules out septic emboli and *myxoma?*

*Pathological Assessment:

– Biopsy to be taken from affected site.
– Biopsy from skin (deep section), nerves and muscle, gallbladder, and appendix biopsies can show a picture of vasculitis if they are inflamed.
– Don't biopsy the kidney as this intervention can lead to intraparenchymal bleeding.

- If biopsy is negative or not accessible and the diagnosis is highly suspected, *negative biopsy will not R/O PAN.*
- Biopsy will show segmental area of necrotizing medium-vessel inflammation with polymorphic neutrophilic infiltration.

*Simplified approach for diagnosis of patients with PAN:

- When the patient is looking sick and has manifestations suggestive of vasculitis in general, the most important step is to rule out infections causing vasculitis mimickers, then

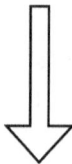

- If vasculitis mimickers have been ruled out, >>> symptoms suspicious for (PAN), the physician should look for: aneurysm by angiography (MRA?), or biopsy from affected site and hepatitis serology.

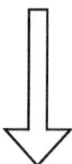

- If not possible to get aforementioned angiogram or biopsy, look for neuropathy with confirmatory tests like EMG/NCS and nerve biopsy, and look for livedo reticularis, testicular pain or tenderness, diastolic BP > 90 mm Hg.

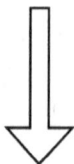

- Be sure that ANCA-associated vasculitis-related symptoms have been searched for comprehensively (EGPA, GPA, and

MPA) as PAN is considered a disease to be diagnosed after exclusion.

*Differential diagnosis in case with PAN:

1– Infectious causes like infective endocarditis or viral.
2– Atherosclerosis: no aneurysms, and conventional digital subtraction angiography is the best test to determine this etiology.
3– Segmental arterial mediolysis: a disease that affects middle-aged to older patients with non-atherosclerotic and noninflammatory pattern associated with degeneration of medial layers in the celiac and mesenteric arterial branches. It causes dissecting aneurysms that spare the bifurcation and leads to life-threatening mesenteric or intraperitoneal hemorrhage.
4– Fibromuscular dysplasia: a condition that is usually affecting young-aged women with aneurismal dilation and *strings on bead* phenotype in angiography. It is predominantly seen in the renal and carotid circulation, and the patient will present with early-onset HTN.
5– Ehler-Danlos syndrome: type IV which is autosomal dominant heritable connective tissue disorder (collagen type III) characterized by aneurismal dilation and rupture of hollow visceral organs. *Genetic testing is necessary!*
6– Malignancies: atrial myxoma or hematological neoplasm.
7– Catastrophic APS: can present with multisystem microthrombi causing multiple organ infarctions.
8– Cholesterol emboli: mainly post vascular intervention.
9– ANCA-associated vasculitis *should be excluded!*

*Clinical phenotypes of PAN:

A- HBV-related PAN (more orchitis, more HTN, or more GI symptoms) versus non-HBV-related PAN.

B- Systemic PAN: associated with systemic symptoms and microaneurysm.

C- Limited cutaneous PAN: subtype presents with ulcerative cutaneous lesions, with some patients that can present with fever. Excisional biopsy is required, and treatment is prednisolone 20 to 40 mg PO once a day, with tapering gradually over two to three months with possibility of adding another immunosuppressive medications like MTX, azathioprine, and rituximab.

D- Single-organ PAN: PAN can involve single organs like gallbladder, appendix, and breast. Surgical excision is the treatment, and the patient needs to be followed.

*Management of PAN:

>>> Identify FFS (proteinuria > 1 g/day, creatinine > 120.5 mcmol/L, cardiomyopathy, GI symptoms, and CNS involvement).

^^ Non HBV-related PAN:

--->If the patient has mild symptoms with joints pain, anemia, and cutaneous lesion with constitutional manifestations (FFS=0), give the patient high dose prednisolone 1 mg/kg per day, tapered over eight to twelve months, and in case of relapse, you can add MTX or azathioprine, with 80 percent achieved remission with steroid alone.

--->If the patient has FFS more than or equal to one, give the patient high dose prednisolone 1 mg/kg per day, tapered gradually over fifteen to eighteen months, and cyclophosphamide (IV NIH protocol) for every two weeks for three doses, then every three weeks for three to four doses (CYCLOPS regimen), followed by maintenance therapy (MTX or azathioprine).

--->*In case of relapsing disease post trial of cyclophosphamide, RTX as lymphoma protocol or anti-TNF like infliximab can be tried.*

--->*Also, IVIG (0.4g/kg daily for five days) can be used to induce remission in case of refractory disease pattern.*

^^HBV-related PAN:

\--->The management should be in collaboration with hepatologist

\--->The treatment is dependent mainly on high dose of steroid (60 mg PO daily), tapered and discontinued rapidly within two weeks. After finishing the course of steroid, initiate PLEX three times weekly for three weeks, then two times weekly for two weeks, then once weekly till seroconversion (HBeAg positive to anti HBeAg) and antiviral medication. This approach achieves seroconversion in about 50 percent, with no relapse in most of the patients.

^^Control BP is paramount (ACEI/CCB).

^^Influenza and pneumococcal vaccines should be administered.

^^Osteoporosis prophylaxis is mandatory.

^^ Age over 50 years at diagnosis and the presence of any factor from FFS system >>> associated with poor prognosis.

^^If the patient has been treated: HBV-related PAN five years survival rate is 73 percent, compared with non-HBV-related PAN at 83 percent.

^^The relapse rate in PAN is lower than in ANCA-associated vasculitis (20 percent) over five years.

^^The cause of death in first year: uncontrolled vasculitic damage and side effects from immunosuppressant.

^^Referral to physiotherapy and rehabilitation is necessary to help the recovery of injured nervous system.

#Monitoring for the patients with PAN: the visit should be arranged earlier every one to three months initially, then every three to six months.

- ^ You should ask the patient about clinical symptoms of PAN.
- ^ Request labs and inflammatory markers.
- ^ Look for complications of PAN: digital ulceration, cardiac failure, renal failure, GI perforation, stroke, seizure, and visual loss.

- Imaging: no need to repeat it unless the patient has an acute and active emergent condition.
- Every visit, you should calculate BVAS, and any score above zero will be considered active disease (BVAS=new symptom).
- Control atherosclerotic risk factors tightly.

*Primary Angiitis of the Central Nervous System (PACNS):
classified as sub type of single organ vasculitis

^ Introduction:

- Rare form of vasculitis affects intracerebral blood vessels.
- More common in men (2:1 M:F), with mean age at diagnosis about fifty years.
- The disease is characterized by indolent course with symptoms appearing over months.

*Pathogenesis:

- PACNS is a disease characterized by peculiar manifestation. The main pathway for occurrence of such inflammation is infiltration of small to medium sized leptomeningeal blood vessels with giant cells or lymphocytes.
- As a result of inflammation, the affected blood vessels will be occluded and causing ischemia and necrosis of the territories of blood vessels.
- The initiating trigger is not well-defined. However, an associated immunosuppressive state leads to abnormal immune vasculitic response.
- There are many infectious agents blamed to be a trigger for vasculitic pathology, like Cytomegalovirus (CMV), human immunodeficiency virus (HIV), and Varicella-Zoster virus (VZV).

*Clinical Assessment:

^ By History:

- You have to ask about history of headache, as it is considered the most common symptom, followed by encephalopathy (cognitive impairment and forgetfulness)
- Recurrent attacks of stroke or TIA (30 to 50 percent) (in absence of atherosclerotic risk factors)
- Seizure
- Behavioral changes

- Ataxia
- Visual changes
- Myelopathy
- Ask about long-standing history of DM, HTN, and dyslipidemia >>> atherosclerosis
- Any symptoms of SLE or Sjogren's syndrome
- History of recurrent thrombosis (APS)
- Ask about risk factors for HIV, syphilis, vesicular rash, and TB
- Any history of immunosuppressive medications use
- Any history of malignancy
- Any illicit drugs use
- Sickle cell disease

>>>Constitutional symptoms are not commonly seen among patients with PACNS.

>>>The onset of PACNS symptoms is insidious and takes a long time to appear (months to years).

^ By Examination:

- Check the vitals: BP is important (acute headache and high BP raise suspicion for reversible cerebral vasoconstriction syndrome).
- Any focal neurological deficit.
- Look for signs of drug injections.

*Proposed Criteria for Primary Angiitis of the Central Nervous System (1988 Calabrese and Mallek proposed diagnostic criteria for PACNS):

- A history of an unexplained neurological deficit,
- With presence of either classical angiographic or histopathological features of angiitis,
- And no evidence of systemic vasculitis or any other condition to which the angiographic or pathologic evidence can be attributed.

>>>Definite diagnosis: when the diagnosis has been supported by biopsy.

CLINICAL NOTES IN VASCULITIC DISEASES

>>>Probable diagnosis: when the diagnosis was done without tissue sample.

*Investigations:

>>>Basic labs:

1– CBC: usually normal.
2– Renal and hepatic profiles: they are normal in case of PACNS.
3– Inflammatory markers: ESR and CRP are *not rising* in PACNS. If they were elevated, think about secondary causes of CNS vasculitis.
4– LDH: RO hematological malignancies (lymphoma especially if elevated more than three times above normal).
5– HIV, hepatitis, CMV, and syphilis serologies.
6– ANA/ANCA mostly are negative.
7– QuantiFERON-TB testing.
8– Hemoglobin electrophoresis.
9– Lumbar Puncture is abnormal in about 80–90 percent, with rise in cells up to 250 with high total protein about 70g/L >>> important to exclude infection.

>>>Basic Imaging:

1– MRI/MRA: 90–100 percent of patients with PACNS have abnormal MRI/MRA with subcortical white matter changes being the most common finding, followed by deep gray matter. If the patient has multiple infarcts bilaterally reported in different intracerebral vascular territories, raise suspicion for (PACNS).
2– Angiogram: abnormal angiogram noted in about 50–90 percent of patients with PACNS, *beading appearance or multiple areas of narrowing* >>> *microaneurysms* are seldom seen.
3– Echocardiogram: to R/O septic emboli.

*Pathological assessment of PACNS:

– All patients with suspected PACNS should be assessed by a neurosurgeon for biopsy.

- To be taken from nondominant temporal lobe and leptomeningeal tissues.
- The sensitivity of tissue biopsy is ranging between 40–50 percent due to nature of the disease *(patchy disease)*.
- There is a study done to test tissue samples from sixty-one patients referred as suspected cases of PACNS. Thirty-nine percent of tissue samples came back with another diagnoses like infections and CNS lymphoma.

*Simplified approach for diagnosis patients with PACNS:

- In case of acute presentation with new onset focal symptom (headache),

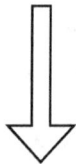

- Do LP and MRI/MRA. If LP results are abnormal, look for infection.

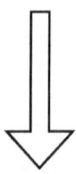

- If LP results are normal with abnormal MRI, proceed for angiogram.

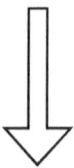

- If angiogram is abnormal, look for vasculitis mimickers (RCVS). But if normal angiogram, try to R/O other etiologies.

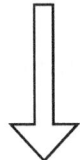

- In case of insidious onset symptoms over months, proceed for LP and MRI/MRA.

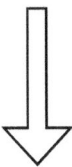

- If LP results are normal with abnormal MRI, proceed for angiography, and in case of abnormal angiogram result, go to biopsy.

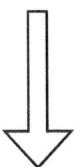

- In case of abnormal CSF analysis, try to find out the causes for chronic meningitis. Then if negative, consider biopsy for PACNS.

★Differential diagnosis in case with PACNS:

^^Mimickers for PACNS:
A-Systemic connective tissue disorders: ★SLE ★Sjogren's syndrome ★PAN ★Sarcoidosis ★ANCA-associated vasculitis ★Behcet's disease

B-Vasculopathies:
*Reversible cerebral vasoconstriction syndrome *Atherosclerosis *Anti phospholipid syndrome *Moyamoya disease *Susac's syndrome (microvasculopathy with corpus collosum involvement, SNHL, and retinal vasculitic disease) *Amphetamine-induced vasospasm
C-Infections:
*Bacterial meningitis *Chronic fungal event *Viral: HIV, varicella *Septic emboli
D-Malignant causes:
*Lymphoma *Leukemia *Lymphomatoid granulomatosis

^^The most important differential diagnosis in case of PACNS is reversible cerebral vasoconstriction syndrome (RCVS).

RCVS	PACNS	Features
More in females	More in males	Gender
Acute	Gradual	Onset
Insidious	Monophasic	Course
Normal/near	Abnormal	CSF findings
100%	50%	Angiogram positive
Calcium channel blocker or steroid?	Steroid and CYC	Treatment
Excellent	Good	Prognosis

*Subtypes of PACNS:

A- *Granulomatous Subtype:* most common form of PACNS, and angiogram in most of the patients is likely to be normal in such cases, and leptomeninges commonly affected. Biopsy is needed.

B- *Lymphocytic Subtype:* second most common subtype of PACNS and very likely to respond to treatment favorably in opposite to other subtypes.

C- *Mass-like subtype:* rare subtype; infectious agents, neoplasia, and amyloidosis should be ruled out by biopsy.

D- *Amyloid B-related angiitis subtype:* more acute in onset in older male patients with cognitive impairment picture and perivascular cell infiltrate.

E- *Angiographically defined subtype:* negative biopsy but abnormal angiogram and CSF analysis.

F- *Spinal cord involvement subtype:* presented with myelopathy picture, negative angiogram, positive MRI/MRA with enhancing lesion (thoracic region), and positive biopsy for necrosis.

*Management of PACNS:

1– Multidisciplinary approach is important in cases of PACNS: rheumatologist, neurologist, neurosurgeon, radiologist, and physiotherapist.
2– The treatment is composed of high dose steroid (1 mg/kg) PO once daily, tapered over three to six 6 months and cyclophosphamide (NIH protocol) for six doses monthly (750 mg/m2 per dose).
3– After the induction phase, the treatment will focus on maintenance immunosuppressive therapies like azathioprine (2 mg/kg per day) or MMF (1–2 g/day). Duration for maintenance therapy ~ two years.
4– In case of refractory or relapsing disease, rituximab can be used, or TNFi (infliximab and etanercept), or tocilizumab, based on case reports with helping improvement or stabilizing the lesion.
5– Osteoporosis prophylaxis or PCP prophylaxis.

*Monitoring:

A- Follow-up to be arranged after four to six weeks from diagnosis, then every four months in the first year, then every three to six months.

B- MRI/MRA to be done regularly to be sure that there is no progression of the disease.

C- The prognosis is good: the mortality rate is 10–15 percent if the patients are being treated *(stroke* is the cause). The relapse rate is ranging between 20–30 percent with presence of seizure at the time of diagnosis, and meningeal enhancement in MRI are major predictors for relapse.

*Thrombangiitis Obliterans (Buerger's Disease):

^Introduction:

- Thrombangiitis obliterans (TAO) is a non-atherosclerotic vasculitic inflammatory disorder affecting small to medium sized blood vessels in the distal extremities.
- The disease occurs mainly in males. However, female patients are reported in about 11–23 percent. TAO is strongly associated with smoking.
- It differs from other types of vasculitis in that patients with TAO are not having any rise in inflammatory markers (ESR, CRP).

★Pathogenesis:

- TAO pathology is complicated, and the process of inflammation occurs due to interaction between different triggers.
- Smoking: It enhances cellular sensitivity to type I or type III collagen and will lead to abnormal vascular reactivity.
- Genetic: Genetic abnormalities in HLA-A9/HLA-B5 can predispose the patients for TAO.
- Endothelial dysfunction: Anti–endothelial cell antibodies been reported among patients with TAO, and these antibodies impair vascular relaxation.
- Infection: Periodontal disease with bacterial pathogens can induce the inflammation *(periodontitis-induced vascular inflammation)*.
- Abnormal immunological response: with presence of anti-cardiolipin antibodies and antibodies against bacterial pathogens. Also, abnormal expression of intracellular adhesion molecule with increase in TNF-a and leukocytes adhesion.

★Clinical Assessment:

^By History:

- You have to ask the patients about symptoms of foot pain.
- Intermittent claudication.
- Any history of rest pain.

- History suggestive of ischemic ulcers or gangrene.
- Migratory superficial thrombophlebitis *(phlebitis saltans)* in 40–60 percent.
- Raynaud's phenomenon can be a manifestation in TAO.
- Joints pain among patients with TAO is seen and mostly affecting wrist and knee joints.
- *History of smoking! Important point.*
- Any history of drug abuse (cocaine or amphetamine).
- Any previous history of recurrent thrombosis (?) for hereditary thrombophilia (?).
- History of malignancy, like lymphoma to R/O cold agglutinin disease?
- Any atherosclerotic risk factors, like DM, HTN, and dyslipidemia.
- Features suggestive for systemic sclerosis (advanced Raynaud's phenomenon).

^By Examination:

- Observe any signs for ischemia (paraesthesia, pulselessness, pain, pallor, paralysis, and cold).
- Look for any digital ulcers.
- Any signs of infection in the wound.
- Assess for peripheral pulses (asymmetry) or any difference in BP.
- Allen's test to examine peripheral vasculature: Ask the patient to do fist many times repetitively, then to do tight fist, and the examiner should press by thumb fingers on ulnar and radial arteries. After that, ask the patient to open the fist and release the pressure on radial artery and check the color of the hand. Then in the next time, release the pressure from ulnar artery.

#Two or more limbs are always affected among patients with TAO.

#The most injured arteries in TAO are anterior and posterior tibial arteries in the lower extremities, and ulnar artery in the upper extremities.

★★Diagnostic criteria by *Olin* for diagnosis (TAO): All of criteria should be met for diagnosing patients with TAO.

1– Onset before age forty-five years,
2– current or recent past history of tobacco use,
3– distal extremity ischemia (claudication, rest pain, ulcers, and gangrene),
4– Laboratory test to exclude autoimmune CTD and diabetes,
5– exclude proximal cause of emboli (echocardiography), and
6– demonstrate consistent arteriographic finding in the involved limbs.

★Investigations:

>>>Basic labs:

1– CBC with differentials: look for high hematocrit or high platelets count >>> R/O myeloproliferative neoplasia (also blood smear is paramount!).
2– Renal (urinalysis and urine toxicology) and liver profiles.
3– Hemoglobin A1c %.
4– Lipid profile.
5– Inflammatory markers (are not significantly rising).
6– ANA and cryoglobulin, rheumatoid factor, and ANCA level >>> R/O vasculitis.
7– Cryofibrinogen and cold agglutinin titer. Those disorders can cause limb ischemia.
8– Anti Scl-70 and anti-centromere antibodies to be requested.
9– Work-up for thrombophilia (aPL antibodies, protein S and C deficiency, prothrombin gene mutation, anti-thrombin III deficiency, and homocysteinemia).

>>>Basic imaging:

1– Ankle-Brachial index (ABI) and wrist-brachial index (WBI) to assess for poor vasculature: If they are negative, it doesn't mean TAO has been ruled out.

2– Duplex Ultrasound for testing blood flow in the blood vessels.

3– Arteriogram (segmental occlusion, no thromboembolic focus, distal arterial involvement, and corkscrew collaterals) is advised to be done in both upper and lower limbs.

4– Echocardiogram: look for any source of emboli.

★Pathological assessment: (Biopsy is rarely required to confirm the diagnosis. However, most of histopathological findings are taken from samples post amputation.)

^   Three pathological phases seen:

A- Acute phase: acute inflammatory response with neutrophils associated with high cellular occlusive thrombus.

B- Intermediate phase: progressive occlusive thrombus with less deposition of inflammatory cells.

C- Chronic phase: occlusive thrombus with extensive recanalization with periadventitial fibrosis.

---->There is no disruption in the architecture of adjacent blood vessels or internal elastic lamina.

★Simplified approach for diagnosis patients with TAO:

- If the patient has symptoms of distal digital ischemia, *poor perfusion,*

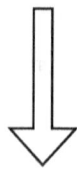

- Take full history and ask specifically about smoking, drug abuse, and other causes of digital ischemia.

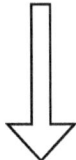

- If no cause apparently seen, proceed to do simple labs to R/O myeloproliferative neoplasia or hereditary thrombophilia.

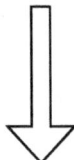

- If all labs turn back negative and no atherosclerotic risk factors,

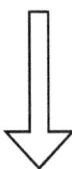

- Proceed for duplex ultrasound, echocardiogram, and arteriogram to confirm diagnosis of TAO.

*Differential diagnosis in case with TAO:

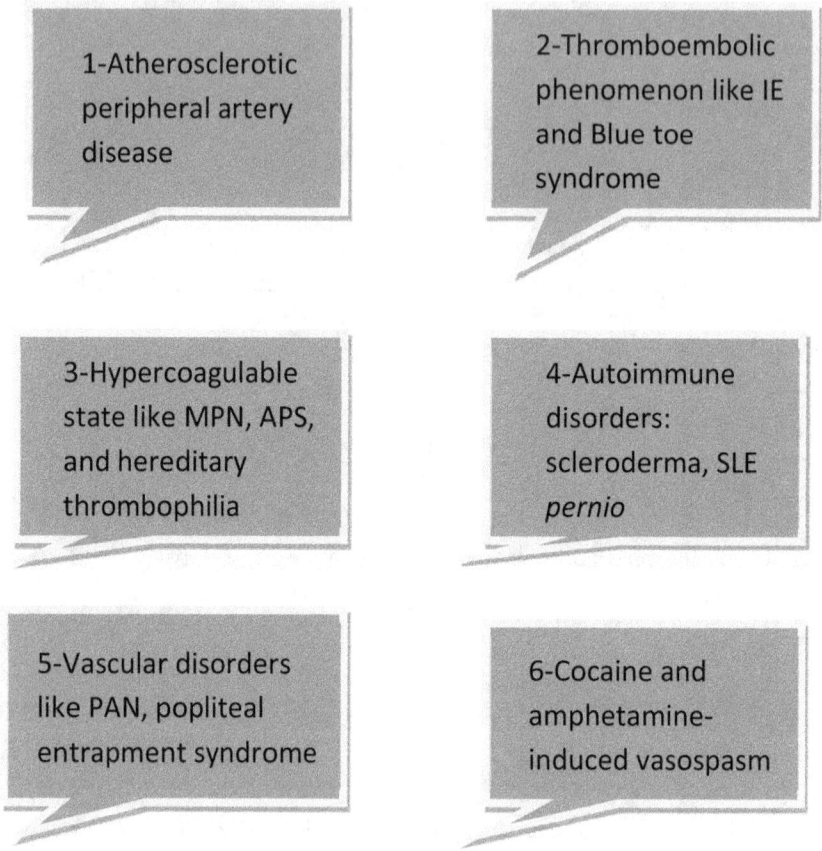

1-Atherosclerotic peripheral artery disease

2-Thromboembolic phenomenon like IE and Blue toe syndrome

3-Hypercoagulable state like MPN, APS, and hereditary thrombophilia

4-Autoimmune disorders: scleroderma, SLE *pernio*

5-Vascular disorders like PAN, popliteal entrapment syndrome

6-Cocaine and amphetamine-induced vasospasm

*Management:

A- *The most important step in management is to advise the patient strongly to discontinue smoking.*

B- *Wound care is important among patients with (TAO), and you should examine if there is any sign of infection for Abx.*

C- Antiplatelets therapies (ASA or clopidogrel): They are not clearly indicated in patients diagnosed with TAO, but possibly beneficial in reducing events associated with atherosclerotic risk factors.

D- Vasodilatory therapies: amlodipine or nifedipine can improve blood flow and increase pain-free walking distance.

E- Ileoprost *vasodilator with decrease in platelets aggregation:* IV administration of prostacyclin analogue in case of ischemia can decrease the pain with improvement in trophic changes based on randomized study.

F- Cilostazol *inhibitor of phosphodiesterase type III:* can increase the level of (cAMP) and enhance vascular relaxation and decrease platelets clumping. (Be careful if the patient developed heart failure to stop it).

G- Intermittent pneumatic compression *IPC:* being shown in the study that IPC can improve wound healing and decreasing the pain.

H- Surgical revascularization is not frequently possible as the disease is segmental and involving arteries in the distal parts of the limb (Consult vascular surgeon!).

*Monitoring:

1– The patient can be followed regularly to be sure that the quality of life is good and not being disturbed.
2– Smoking cessation is extremely important to improve the symptoms and decrease the need for amputation.
3– Based on one study, 34 percent of the patients with TAO will experience one amputation in fifteen years after diagnosis.
4– *Non-white patients and limb infection at the time of diagnosis* were independently associated with more vascular events.

*Kawasaki Disease (KD):

^ Introduction:

- Kawasaki disease is a type of small to medium vessels vasculitis that occur predominantly among children with age < five years.
- It affects more patients from Asian descent (rate 29.8 per 100,000 with males more affected).
- The diagnosis is dependent on clinical picture, with lab results indicative for inflammation.

*Pathogenesis:

- The pathology in Kawasaki disease is poorly understood. However, the interaction between genetic, infectious, and abnormal immune regulation may play a role.
- Genetic background is released from an evidence that increased risk of Kawasaki disease among identical twins is 13 percent.
- Single-nucleotide polymorphism (SNP) in different genes blamed as a trigger for (KD), such as caspase-3 and B-cell lymphoid kinase.
- Unknown infectious trigger may be a factor that can activate immune system, like adenovirus?
- Seasonality phenomenon may be a good theory that can explain KD is more prevalent during the month of January, with another peak from spring to summer.
- Dysregulated innate immune response with detection of pathogen-associated molecular pattern (PAMP) leads to activation of (NLRP3) inflammasome that can propagate the production of cascade of inflammatory cytokines like IL-1, IL-6, IL-8, IL-18, IFN-gamma, and TNF-a.
- As a result of activation of innate immune system, adaptive immune system will be stimulated. There is an increment in number of circulating T-regulatory cells and enhanced number of IgA-producing plasma cells.

>>>The production of inflammatory cytokines with stimulation of T and B cells will induce tissue inflammation (e.g., coronaries).

CLINICAL NOTES IN VASCULITIC DISEASES

★Clinical assessment:

- By History:
- Ask about history of prolonged unexplained fever (temp. >39 C) for seven to fourteen days.
- Ask about eye symptoms *(conjunctivitis)* which are non-purulent, limbic sparing, and bilateral.
- Also, you have to be aware about any oral mucosal changes or any cracking of the lips.
- Look for any diffuse erythematous rash.
- Observe for diffuse swelling of the hands with peeling of the skin.

-By Examination:

- Check the vitals: fever? BP, tachycardia, or tachypnea.
- Irritable child due to fever; *aseptic meningitis* is a possibility!
- Examine for oral mucosal redness, *strawberry tongue*.
- Look for cervical lymphadenopathy (unilateral).
- Signs of heart failure (volume overload).
- GI examination (RUQ tenderness) >>> gallbladder hydrops.

★★Diagnostic criteria for Kawasaki disease (KD):

1– Mucosal changes: erythema and cracking of the lips, or erythema of pharyngeal mucosa.
2– Conjunctivitis: bilateral bulbar, non-purulent conjunctival injection.
3– Polymorphous rash: maculopapular, diffuse erythematous rash.
4– Extremity changes: erythema and edema of hands and feet with desquamation.
5– Lymphadenopathy: more than or equal to 1.5 cm unilateral cervical LN enlargement.

>>The patient must have more than or equal to five days of fever, with more than or equal four out of five features present in the criteria.

**Less common features seen in patients with Kawasaki disease (KD):

-Cardiovascular:
Myocarditis or pericarditis
Valvular regurgitation
Aortic root enlargement

-Respiratory:
Pleural effusion
Empyema
Interstitial infiltrate in chest radiograph

-Gastrointestinal:
Vomiting or Diarrhea
Gallbladder hydrops
Pancreatitis

-Nervous system:
Aseptic meningitis
CVA
Behavioral changes or irritability

-Genitourinary:
Urethritis
Hydrops

-Eye:
Anterior uveitis by slit lamp examination

KAWASAKI DISEASE
Triphasic

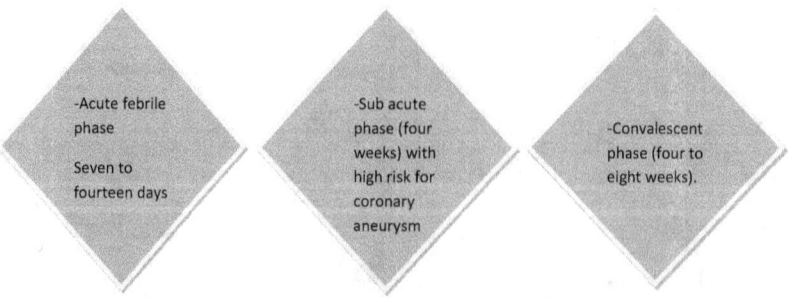

- Acute febrile phase — Seven to fourteen days
- Sub acute phase (four weeks) with high risk for coronary aneurysm
- Convalescent phase (four to eight weeks).

*Investigations:

>>>Basic labs:

- CBC with differentials: anemia of chronic disease and thrombocytosis with high platelets count up to 1,000,000 per mm3 in the first week post symptoms in patients with KD.
- Renal and liver profiles: serum transaminases and GGT are elevated in 40–60 percent of patients with KD. Also, hypoalbuminemia being noticed in KD.
- Urinalysis: sterile pyuria seen in up to 80 percent of affected children with KD.
- Acute phase reactants (elevated): ESR > 40 mm/hr and CRP > 3g/dl.
- Viral work-up to be ordered: EBV, measles, HIV, and adenovirus.
- Blood culture: to R/O bacteremia (staphylococcal toxic shock syndrome).

>>>Don't forget to request COVID-19 swab as this infection is being blamed to cause Kawasaki disease-like syndrome.

>>>Basic imaging:

- Echocardiography: to assess cardiac function and valvular abnormalities or examine for coronary artery lesions (Z-score=dimensions of coronary artery adjusted for body surface area).
- Cardiac MR: to look for any structural defects. Chest X-ray to see if there is any infiltrate.

Risk Factors for developing coronary artery lesions (CAL):
A-Age less than one year or more than eight years
B-Anemia < 10 g/dl, thrombocytopenia, leukocytosis > 15
C-Hypoalbuminemia and hyponatremia
D-Persistent fever of more than ten days
E-Recurrence of fever thirty-six hours post IVIG administration

*Simplified approach for diagnosis patients with KD:

- If the child has persistent spikes of fever with sick appearance,

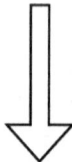

- Try to rule out comprehensively the cause of this fever such as infectious causes.

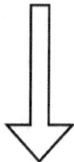

- If all causes been excluded, you can request basic labs indicative for general inflammation and look for what is called *incomplete Kawasaki disease* (by expert physician).

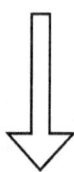

>> Always try to exclude *macrophage activation syndrome* as it is fatal if not caught early.

CLINICAL NOTES IN VASCULITIC DISEASES

★Differential diagnosis in case with KD:

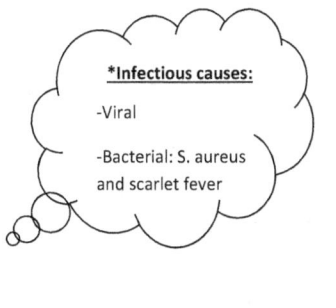

*Infectious causes:
- Viral
- Bacterial: S. aureus and scarlet fever

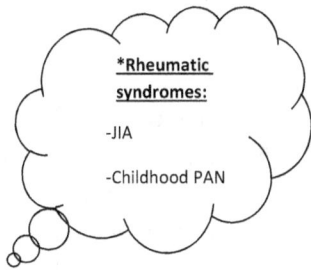

*Rheumatic syndromes:
- JIA
- Childhood PAN

*Drugs-related:
- Drug hypersensitivity syndrome

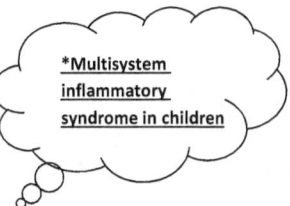

*Multisystem inflammatory syndrome in children

*Multisystem inflammatory syndrome in children
MIS-C

A- New entity being discovered in the era of COVID-19 as a result of cytokines-induced inflammation (post COVID by four weeks).

B- Age of the patient is more than five years and less than twenty-one years.

C- Multi organs involvement and high markers of inflammation and required hospitalization.

Question: Can Kawasaki disease occur in adult patients?

^ It can occur rarely after exclusion of different causes, like infections, malignancy, and other autoimmune disorders.
^ There are some cases reported to have Kawasaki disease in adults.
^ We have to exclude HIV. It is very important!
^ Adult patients with Kawasaki disease (KD) tend to have more cervical lymphadenopathy, hepatitis, and arthralgia. The occurrence of coronary artery aneurysms and thrombocytosis are less frequent among adult patients.
^ Treatment: same as in children, (IVIG) and Acetylsalicylic acid (ASA).

*Management:

A- Early administration of (IVIG) is extremely important in Kawasaki disease, as its early initiation will be associated with reduction of the risk for coronary artery lesions from 25 percent to 3–5 percent *(initiation* with ten days of fever).

B- The dose of (IVIG) is 2 g/kg to be given initially over ten to twelve hours. There are some children (20 percent) who will have recurrent or persistent fever >>> IVIG-resistant patients.

C- Risk factors for IVIG resistance: delayed administration of IVIG, cervical lynphadenopathy, oral mucosal changes, decreased hemoglobin and platelets, elevated ESR, and diffuse extremity swelling. It is recommended to give those patients another dose of IVIG to prevent complications.

D- Acetylsalicylic acid (ASA) should be given in combination with IVIG with moderate dose (30–50 mg/kg/day divided every six hours during acute febrile phase). Then after the fever subsided, switch the patients into low dose (3–5 mg/kg/day) for its antiplatelets effect. ASA should be continued for six to eight weeks, and after this period, the plan about continuing this therapy is dependent on coronary artery lesions formation.

E- Regarding corticosteroid therapy: most of vasculitic cases respond very well to steroid therapy. Its use among patients with Kawasaki disease (KD) has conflict. A meta-analysis showed that early initiation of steroid and IVIG/ASA since the beginning was associated with lower incidence of coronary artery lesions in comparison to delayed initiation of steroid post IVIG. Until now, there is no clear recommendation about initiation of steroid in Kawasaki disease. However, its use in patient with positive risk factors for IVIG resistance can be considered. The dose is about 1–6 mg/kg/day for longer duration of more than three days.

F- In cases of IVIG resistance Kawasaki disease, use of TNFi like INFLIXIMAB in one single dose 5 *mg/kg* is advised, as it will decrease the duration of fever and decrease the duration of hospitalization.

G- Use of other agents among patients with IVIG resistance like *cyclosporin* is beneficial as it will decrease the risk of coronary artery lesions. Also, IL-1i use, such as *anakinra*, can be a valid option among patients with refractory disease.

H- Tocilizumab (IL-6i) is not used in management of KD, although IL-6 is involved in pathogenesis of KD. This drug can cause progressive development of giant coronary aneurysm based on case series.

~~*The involvement of pediatric cardiologist in management of patients with KD is strongly advised.*

★★The use of antiplatelets in patients without coronary artery lesions should be continued for six to eight weeks.

^^Patients with small-sized coronary artery lesion of less than 5 mm can be continued on ASA monotherapy, while medium-sized coronary artery lesion to be on combined ASA and clopidogrel.

##Children affected with KD and have large coronary artery lesion of more than 8 mm can be continued on combined antiplatelets and anticoagulant.

**Monitoring:

1– Echocardiography should be done at the time of diagnosis, then to be repeated after two weeks, and later to be repeated six to eight weeks from the first time of diagnosis to decide about any development of coronary artery lesions.
2– The recurrence rate of Kawasaki disease is less than 3 percent. So, it is advisable to ask the patients about symptoms of KD in each visit.
3– There is an important thing we have to consider post IVIG therapy: live vaccines, such as measles and varicella, should be delayed for eleven months post IVIG dose.
4– Follow-up with pediatric cardiologist is important to have a clear plan about coronary artery lesions and the need for antiplatelets therapy. The patients with coronary artery lesions with enlarged aneurysm should have close monitoring.
5– The most common cause of death among patients with KD is myocardial infarction secondary to coronary artery occlusion. It is better to explain to the family about this complication.
6– Don't forget to request antibodies against COVID-19 in patients presenting with Kawasaki disease-like illness (MIS-C).

*SMALL VESSELS VASCULITIS:

-Immune complex mediated small vessels vasculitis:

^Anti-glomerular basement membrane (anti-GBM) disease

^IgA vasculitis (HSP)

^Cryoglobulinemic vasculitis (CV)

^Hypocomplementemic urticarial vasculitis (HUVS)

-Antineutrophilic cytoplasmic antibody ANCA-associated vasculitis:

^Granulomatosis with polyangiitis (GPA)

^Microscopic polyangiitis (MPA)

^Eosinophilic granulomatosis with polyangiitis (EGPA)

CLINICAL NOTES IN VASCULITIC DISEASES

*IgA vasculitis (Henoch-Schonlein Purpura):

^ Introduction:

- It is the most common subtype of systemic vasculitis in children. It affects children with age of less than ten years, with slight male predominance (M:F ratio = 1.5).
- It involves small blood vessels (arteriole, capillary, and venules), and occurs frequently during winter and fall seasons.
- It is characterized by presence of palpable purpura, abdominal pain, and articular symptoms. GI and renal involvement can happen and leads to devastating complications.

★Pathogenesis:

- IgA (IgA1> IgA 2) is the most prominent subclass of immunoglobulin found in mucosal areas.
- It is participating in mucosal defense, killing and agglutinating the microbes.
- Healthy IgA should have proper N-acetylgalactosamine (GaINAc) binding. However, when IgA1 will have deficiency in galactose, this will promote immune complex formation by production of IgG against IgA with lack in galactose.
- Genetic background may have an impact on occurrence of IgA vasculitis. Variants of HLA-B1★01 and HLA-B1★11 were associated with development of IgA vasculitis.
- Also, infectious triggers like *viral influenza,* S. aureus, and group B streptococci are thought to be inducers for vasculitis by either stimulation of anti-endothelial cell antibodies or by encouraging reactivity between IgG and galactose deficient IgA1.
- The occurrence of small vessels inflammation is promoted by deposition of IgA1 with increased level of anti-endothelial cells antibodies. Additionally, there is rising in *TNF, IL-8, and* Leukotriens (LTB) which will lead to neutrophilic chemoattraction, and as a sequela for this process, vasculitis will occur.

*Clinical assessment:

-By History:

- Ask about any recent history of upper respiratory tract infection or recent drug use.
- Ask about symptoms of cutaneous rash, *painless palpable purpuric rash 96–100 percent* that occurs predominantly in the lower extremities.
- Ask about symptoms of migratory joints pain and swelling, *mainly knee and ankle joints at 61 percent.*
- Don't forget to identify if the patients have any abdominal pain, hematemesis, or hematochezia. *GI involvement is at 48–53 percent and occurs about one week post rash.*
- Ask about any hematuria or frothy urine. *Kidney involvement is at 33–50 percent and usually is developing in about four weeks from onset of disease.*
- Identify any rare complications: neurological symptoms like seizure, headache, and focal neurological deficit. Also, fever and fatigue are common.
- Is there any history of testicular pain and swelling, *orchitis with IgAV?*

-By Examination:

- Check the vitals (high blood pressure >>> renal involvement?).
- Check growth charts.
- Do full GI examination! R/O intussusceptions, GI hemorrhage, and you can do genital examination to see if there is any orchitis.
- Check lower limbs rash (palpable or nonpalpable?). Is there any necrotic lesion or not? The rash could be seen in the lower parts of the arms!
- Check lower limbs edema for renal involvement.
- Do MSK examination! R/O synovitis *(non-deforming arthritis).*

CLINICAL NOTES IN VASCULITIC DISEASES

*Investigations:

>>>Basic labs:

- CBC with differentials and peripheral smear to check for thrombocytopenia (ITP to be excluded).
- Renal profile and urinalysis: any rise in creatinine or drop in eGFR or proteinuria or hematuria (also with twenty-four-hour urine protein collection and send for urine toxicology).
- Liver profile and coagulation profile (if coagulation is being disturbed, look for alternative diagnosis).
- Fecal occult blood or fecal calprotectin >>> unseen GI involvement.
- Immunoglobulin level (IgA will rise in ~ 80 percent). High IgA predicts development of renal disease.
- Blood culture R/O bacteremia as the cause for purpura.
- Request hepatitis A, B, and C serology. Also HIV, QuantiFERON-TB, and Helicobacter pylori checkup should be ordered.

Diagnostic Criteria for IgA Vasculitis from the European League Against Rheumatism and the Pediatric Rheumatology European Society: (Se .99 percent and Sp .86 percent)

>>Mandatory criterion: purpura or petechiae with lower limbs predominance and minimum of one or more of the following:

A-Acute arthritis or arthralgia	B-Diffuse acute abdominal pain
C-Renal involvement	D-Leukocytoclastic vasculitis with IgA deposit or proliferative GN with IgA deposit

- ANA and ds-DNA antibodies to be requested: R/O SLE!
- ANCA and cryoglobulin and complements profiles to be done.

>>>Basic imaging:

- Abdominal X-Ray (erect and supine): signs of obstruction.
- Chest X-Ray (CXR): pulmonary infiltrate >>> *pulmonary hemorrhage is extremely rare in patients with IGA vasculitis (HSP).*
- Abdominal ultrasound: look for intussusceptions.

- KUB-ultrasound to assess renal parenchyma and to assess before going to biopsy.
- CT abdomen and pelvis: look for acute abdomen (GI perforation or obstruction!).
- Upper and lower GI endoscopy: ulcer formation in the small intestine, multiple erythematous lesions seen in the mucosal surfaces of stomach and large intestine.
- Echocardiogram: septic emboli to be excluded.

Pathological assessment:

Skin (leukocytoclastic vasculitis and IgA deposit), or renal (mesangial proliferative GN and IgA deposit), or GI biopsy: to detect vasculitic lesions and IgA deposition in IF assay.

*Simplified approach for diagnosis on patients with HSP:

- In case of patients presented with palpable purpura or abdominal pain,

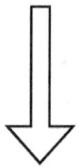

- Ask in the history fully about other symptoms of HSP, and ask about any history suggestive for infection or coagulopathy.

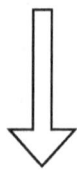

- Request all labs to R/O other types of vasculitis and SLE. Also, you have to R/O infections and hematological disorders (like low platelets!).

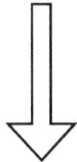

- Other differentials being excluded, we can consider it (HSP vasculitis per criteria) and we can assess the burden of disease.

*Differential diagnosis in case with IgA vasculitis (HSP):

#*Infectious causes:*
- **Bacterial endocarditis**
- **Meningococcemia**
- **Chronic EBV infection**
- **Post-streptococcal disease**

#*Other autoimmune disorders:*
- **ANCA-associated vasculitis**
- **Cryoglobulinemic vasculitis**
- **Hypocomplementemic urticarial vasculitis (HSP can present with urticaria!)**
- **SLE**

#*Hematological disorders:*
- **Immune-thrombocytopenic purpura (ITP)**
- **Thrombotic thrombocytopenic purpura (TTP)**
- **Chronic DIC**
- **Leukemia or lymphoma**

**Patients with IgA vasculitis may present with low factor XIII, especially in patients with GI manifestation.*

**Patients with IgA vasculitis with renal involvement at 10–30 percent will have progressive kidney disease over long term follow-up.*

*Management:

1. We have to identify the extent of disease: cutaneous only or associated with GI or renal abnormalities.
2. Multidisciplinary team approach with gastroenterologist and nephrologist.
3. The course of IgA vasculitis is benign and self-limited, with spontaneous resolution noticed in *children 94 percent and adults 89 percent.*

In case of arthralgia and rash (rest and analgesia recommended >>> NSAIDs can be used).

4. The indications for corticosteroids use in IgA vasculitis: *diffuse purpuric rash, diffuse and severe abdominal pain; significant debilitating arthritis & proteinuria > 1 g/day after three months trial of ACEI/ARB.*
5. *Management of renal involvement among patients with IgA vasculitis*

(IgA nephropathy)

- *Patients with low-risk profile: minor abnormalities in urinalysis, eGFR normal, and **no** hypertension. Monitor the patients annually for ten years.*
- *Moderate to high-risk profile:- proteinuria 500 mg to 1g/day, eGFR reduced and/or hypertension. We have to initiate proper supportive therapy like ACEI to control high blood pressure and avoid salt intake and maintain good fluid balance.*

>>>*Do monitor every three to six months and try to maximize supportive measures. But if proteinuria level > 1 g/day, there is persistent decline in eGFR. Adding corticosteroid is advised.*

- *In case of RPGN or nephrotic syndrome associated with IgA nephropathy or IgA vasculitis:* steroid and immunosuppression should be initiated.

6. Regarding immunosuppressive agents used for renal and non-renal manifestations:

#*Rituximab (RTX):* Anti-CD20 medication that can deplete pathogenic antibodies and prevent T-cell stimulation by B cells. Based on one study, RTX initiated among patient with refractory IgA vasculitis that showed high remission rate of 91 percent with reduction in proteinuria. It can be used either as the disease is refractory or in relapsing phenomenon.

#*Mycophenolate Mofetil (MMF):* It has been studied that MMF *2–3g/day* and low dose prednisolone *0.4–0.5 mg/kg/day* can induce remission among patients with IgA nephropathy-IgA vasculitis and decrease the relapse rate.

#*Cyclosporine A (CsA):* It can be used in combination with steroid for treating *nephrotic syndrome* among patients with IgA nephropathy, and also among patients with bowel perforation as per case reports.

#*Azathioprine:* Its use in adult patients with IgA vasculitis is not supported. However, it can be used as a sparing agent in cutaneous and articular manifestations.

#*Cyclophosphamide (CYC):* There is no strong evidence that encourages the use of cyclophosphamide among patient with IgA vasculitis with either renal or GI involvement. It doesn't alter the prognosis of disease in comparison with steroid alone.

>>>Other less commonly used modalities like:

A- IVIG (also intramuscular form can be used) and the dose 0.35ml/kg intramuscular weekly for four weeks, then every two weeks for thirty-two weeks. This regimen showed improvement in proteinuria, abdominal pain, purpura, and arthritis. This regimen to be used when eGFR>70ml/min and mild to moderate proteinuria.

B- *PLEX:* PLEX administered concomitantly with steroid may induce improvement in proteinuria and eGFR, and decrease the relapse rate after follow-up for ~ six years.

C- *Cryoprecipitate*: As per case reports among pediatric patients, the replacement of factor XIII by cryoprecipitate administration can successfully ameliorate severe GI and renal manifestations among patients with IgA vasculitis (HSP).

D- *Dapsone and Colchicine:* can be tried in patients with relapsing cutaneous disease in IgA vasculitis (HSP).

E- As leukotrienes play a role in pathogenesis of IgA vasculitis, the addition of *Montelukast* in pediatric patients (leukotriene receptor antagonist) to standard therapy may attenuate cutaneous, gastrointestinal, articular symptoms, and decrease proteinuria and hematuria.

---

*Monitoring:

1-The patients can be followed monthly for three months, then every three to six months to be sure about any development of renal or GI complications.

2-The follow-up visit should include: checking the symptoms, checking BP, and checking renal function and urinalysis.

3-Immunosuppressive therapies' side effects should be checked, especially steroid.

4-Ask the patients about any renal, GI, genital, and neurological symptoms in each visit.

*CRYOGLOBULINEMIC VASCULITIS (CryoVas):

*Introduction:

- It is a subtype of small to medium sized vessels vasculitis affecting skin, nervous system, joints, and kidneys.
- Cryoglobulinemia: detection of protein precipitate composed of immunoglobulins accumulated together at cold temperature of 4°C during seven days and dissolved when heated at 37°C (from serum only).
- It may occur as a result of underlying etiology or may manifest in idiopathic manner *(essential* CryoVas).
- Viral hepatitis C (hep. C) is responsible about occurrence of CryoVas in majority of cases.
- It is predominantly seen more among women (2–3:1), with mean age of forty-five to sixty-five years.

*Pathogenesis:

- Immunoglobulins are released after stimulation of B cells to fight against different pathogens.
- When B cells chronically stimulated by longstanding triggers like hepatitis C. Clonal expansion of B cells will occur with abnormal production of immunoglobulin.
- As a result of that, abnormal immune complex deposition will happen with activation of complements pathway. Then inflammation of blood vessels will appear.

**Types of cryoglobulinemic vasculitis (CryoVas):

A-Type I *10–15 percent:* single monoclonal immunoglobulins always linked to B cells lymphoproliferative disorder like Woldenstrom macroglobulinemia.

B-Type II *50–60 percent:* polyclonal IgG with monoclonal IgM with rheumatoid factor activity. This phenomenon is caused mainly by infection and underlying autoimmune CTD.

C-Type III *20–25 percent:* polyclonal IgG with polyclonal IgM with rheumatoid factor activity.
    (Type II or Type III called mixed cryoglobulinemic vasculitis)

*Clinical assessment :-

-By History:

- Ask about any history of purpuric skin rash (lower extremities and abdomen).
- Ask if there is any history of constitutional symptoms like fever, myalgia, night sweating, and weight loss.
- Any history of hyperviscosity symptoms like headache, stroke-like, and vision blurriness (important for plasma cells dyscrasias).
- Any history of Raynaud's phenomenon, digital ulcerations, or gangrene.
- Don't forget to ask about shortness of breath or hemoptysis.
- Ask about any history of autoimmune CTD: sicca symptoms (Sjogren's syndrome), arthritis (RA), oral or nasal ulcers, or malar rash (SLE).
- Any history of foot or wrist drop *(weakness!)*.
- Any history indicative for paraesthesia or numbness.
- Is there any GI symptom like abdominal pain or bleeding per rectum?
- Is there any history of CNS symptom like seizure or cranial neuropathies?
- History of hematuria or frothy urine?
- Any recent medications use.
- Any risk factors for hepatitis C or HIV, blood transfusion, and sexual contact?

-By Examination:

- Check the vitals (temperature or BP).
- Examine for any chest crepitations (R/O pulmonary hemorrhage) or heart murmurs (R/O endocarditis).
- Don't forget to do MSK examination, synovitis!
- GIT examination including digital rectal examination.
- Neurological examination, weakness or decreased sensation.
- Observe for any purpuric rash, necrosis, ulcers, gangrenous digits, and livedo reticularis.

> #Meltzer's Triad: Palpable Purpura, Weakness, and Arthralgia
>
> \>\>This triad is found in most of the patients with mixed CryoVas.

*Proposed classification criteria for diagnosis cryoglobulinemic vasculitis (CryoVas): This criterion includes three domains (questionnaire, clinical, and laboratory), two positive domains, or three considered (CryoVas): *Sensitivity=89 percent and specificity=90–96 percent"*

First Domain *Questionnaire*: two of three questions. This domain will be positive.

- Do you remember one or more episodes of small red spots on your skin, particularly lower limbs?
- Have you ever had red spots on your lower extremities which have brownish color after disappearance?
- Has a doctor ever told you that you have viral hepatitis?

Second Domain *Clinical*: three out of four. This domain will be positive.

- Constitutional symptoms: fatigue, fibromyalgia, low-grade fever, and fever of more than 38°C.
- Articular involvement: arthralgia or arthritis.
- Vascular involvement: purpura, skin ulcers, necrosis, and Raynaud's phenomenon.
- Neurological involvement: peripheral neuropathy, cranial neuropathy, vasculitis nervous system disease.

Third Domain *Laboratory*: two out of three. This domain will be positive.

- Reduced serum level of C4.
- Positive serum rheumatoid factor (RF).
- Positive serum M component.

\>\>\>*Serum cryoglobulin level should be repeated for second time* (twelve weeks apart).

**Frequent conditions associated with development of cryoglobulins:

-Infectious causes:

Hepatitis C: *Most common infection associated with cryoglobulinemia*

HIV

Hepatitis B

Brucella

Coxiella burnetii (Q fever in patients with endocarditis, cryoglobulinemia, and negative culture)

Pulmonary TB

Parvovirus B19

CMV/EBV

-Autoimmune connective tissue disorders:

Sjogren's syndrome

SLE

Rheumatoid arthritis

Systemic sclerosis

-Malignant disorders:

- *Hematological*: Multiple myeloma, Waldenstrom macroglobulinemia, CLL, CML, and B cells lymphoma
- *Other solid malignancies*: Hepatocellular carcinoma, thyroid cancer, renal cell carcinoma, and nasopharyngeal carcinoma

*Investigations:

>>>Basic labs:

- CBC with differentials: anemia or pseudo-thrombocytosis and pseudo-leukocytosis can happen in CryoVas.
- Peripheral smear and LDH level: R/O any abnormal malignant cells *(leukemic cells!)*
- Renal profile, urinalysis, and twenty-four-hour urine protein collection: high creatinine (AKI), hematuria, abnormal urine cast, or proteinuria.
- Liver profile: high transaminase enzymes for hepatitis.
- Complete viral hepatitis serology.
- HIV serology
- QuantiFERON-TB
- Brucella serology
- Blood culture: R/O bacteremia.
- Serum and urine protein electrophoresis: R/O plasma cells dyscrasias,
- ANA, ds-DNA antibodies, anti-SSA or anti-SSB, and rheumatoid factor (RF significant rise in RF is important to diagnose CryoVas).
- Complements (C3 and C4): both of them will be low, but C4 will have preferentially low level.
- Cryoglobulin level: to collect the sample from the patient at room temperature (37°C), then allow for clot at same temperature. After that, the sample will undergo for centrifugation and refrigeration at 4°C for one to seven days. If cryoglobulins are present, it will be at the bottom of the tube. The labs can measure *cryocrit* and *cryoglobulin concentration*.
- If cryoglobulins are present, request for immunofixation to identify the nature of immunoglobulins.
- EMG or nerve conduction study: to recognize any neuropathy *mononeuritis multiplex or asymmetrical polyneuropathy, then it may become symmetrical.*

>>>Basic imaging:

- CT chest, abdomen, and pelvis: to identify if there is any pulmonary hemorrhage, any mass or lymph node enlargement, or mesenteric ischemia.
- Ultrasound kidneys and liver: any hepatomegaly or increased renal echogenicity.

---

*Pathological assessment: (three sites to take biopsy from)

^ Skin: Leukocytoclastic vasculitis involving arterioles, capillaries, and venules (non-specific)
^ Nerves: Vasculitic lesions in vasa vasorum or thrombi in endoneural vessels
^ Kidneys: Membranoproliferative glomerulonephritis with hyaline thrombi in the small blood vessels in the glomeruli

---

*Simplified approach for diagnosis patient with CryoVas:

- If you have one patient who has history of purpura on and off, arthralgia, and fatigue,

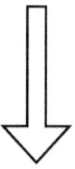

- You have to ask the patient full questions present in the criteria for diagnosis (CryoVas).

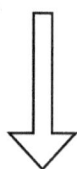

- If the patient answered the questions present in the criteria, now try to R/O chronic infection like hepatitis C, chronic autoimmune CTD, and malignancy, especially lymphoma and hepatocellular carcinoma.

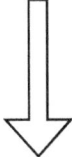

- If no reasons identified and cryoglobulins detected, you can consider it as essential (CryoVas) and continue work-up to have an idea about extent of disease. Does the patient have any major organ involvement?

*Differential diagnosis in case with CryoVas:

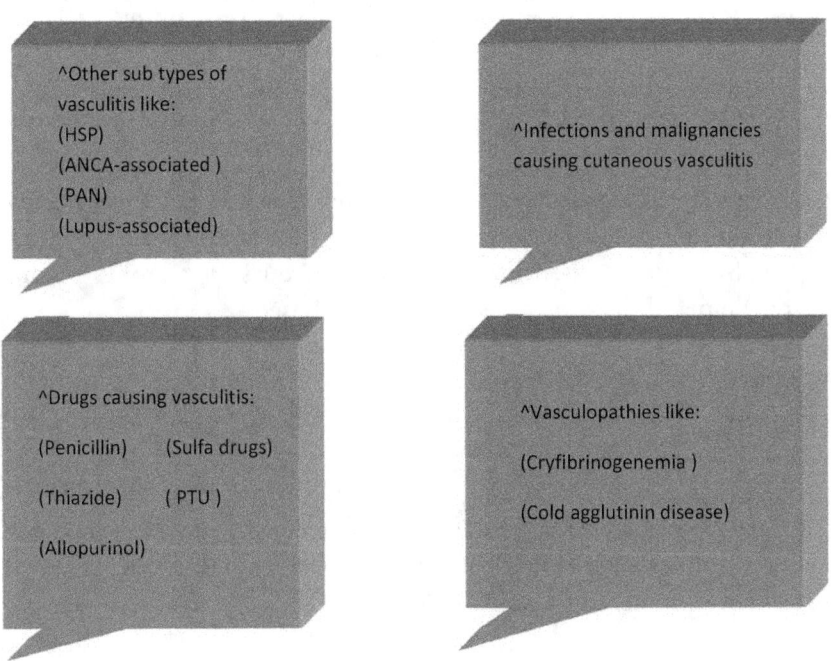

*Management:

1– The treatment plan should be arranged in cooperation with hepatologist or hematologist, dependent on underlying etiology.
2– The aim of treatment is (A) to remove the trigger responsible for production of cryoglobulins, and (B) to control the symptoms of vasculitis.
3– The decision about the medications used is dependent on if the patient has positive hepatitis C serology, and evaluation of the extent of disease. Is there any major organs involvement that is affecting the stability of the patients?
4– In case of cryoglobulinemic vasculitis (CryoVas) with positive serology of hepatitis C, the initiation of direct antiviral therapy is advised based on *vasculvaldic* trial that examined *sofosbuvir and ribavirin* in twenty-four patients diagnosed with HCV-associated cryoglobulinemic vasculitis. At twenty-four weeks, 87.5 percent of the patients achieved complete clinical improvement in all vasculitic symptoms.
5– To classify the manifestations of cryoglobulinemic vasculitis:

*Mild: Arthralgia or arthritis, purpuric rash, and mild paraesthesia, the treatment consists of antiviral therapy if hepatitis C serology is positive +\- low dose prednisolone tapered over a short period. If the patient doesn't have positive hepatitis C serology, a course of steroid (0.5 mg/kg/day) tapered over four to six weeks is advised.

*Moderate: Digital gangrene, cutaneous ulceration, debilitating peripheral neuropathy, and proteinuria or hematuria, the treatment will include antiviral therapy, if hepatitis C serology positivity is documented, steroid (1mg/kg/day) and rituximab therapy *RTX* (either RA or lymphoma protocol). Remission is achieved in about 83 percent in *RTX group*. While in patients without positive hepatitis C serology, treatment will include *steroid and RTX*.

*Severe: Alveolar hemorrhage, RPGN or nephrotic syndrome, myocardial involvement, GI involvement like ischemia, and CNS involvement. The treatment in these organ-threatening conditions should include *steroid* pulse therapy for three days, followed by 1 mg/

kg/day steroid and RTX. The addition of plasma exchange (three sessions per week for two to three weeks) in such cases may be reasonable to remove circulating immune complex. In severe cases with positive hepatitis C serology, the addition of antiviral drugs should be later after induction of remission with immunosuppressive therapies.

6– The use of cyclophosphamide among cases diagnosed with CryoVas can be valuable option among cases refractory to antiviral drugs or RTX.

7– Mycophenolate mofetil (MMF) successfully used to treat CryoVas, especially in patients who have cryoglobulinemia secondary to systemic sclerosis and Sjogren's syndrome.

8– Treatment of Type I cryoglobulinemic vasculitis with hyperviscosity syndrome should be tailored in collaboration with a hematologist. PLEX, steroid, +\- RTX, or other proteasome inhibitor can be considered.

---

*Prognosis of Cryoglobulinemic Vasculitis:

-Among patients with HCV (positive)-related CryoVas:

Five years survival rate = 75 percent, and ten years survival rate = 63 percent

(Poor prognostic factor = presence of severe liver fibrosis, positive FFS)

-Among patients without positive HCV serology:

Five years survival rate = 79 percent, and ten years survival = 65% percent

(Poor prognostic factors = age more than 60 years, renal, GI, and pulmonary involvement)

^^Renal failure is the most common cause of death followed by infection, vasculitis flare, and cardiovascular disease.

*Monitoring:

- RTX is a safe immunosuppressive medication even in case of chronic hepatitis C infection.
- RTX infusion is sometimes associated with infusion reaction, so be careful about this side effect.
- You can give RTX like RA protocol, then every six months (for two years) to prevent relapse with following the patients.
- Ask the patients in each visit about symptoms of major organs involvement with checking blood pressure, urinalysis, and kidney function. Some experts recommend requesting cryoglobulin and rheumatoid factor levels to evaluate the response of therapy.
- You can use Birmingham Vasculitis Activity Score (BVAS) to assess disease response. However, you can evaluate skin ulcer, sensory function, and absence of renal parameters of inflammation to decide about good response of therapy.
- Vaccination is important (influenza and pneumococcal vaccines). Even COVID-19 vaccine can be administered before the dose of RTX by four weeks.

===

*Hypocomplementemic Urticarial Vasculitis Syndrome (HUVS):

★Introduction:

- Urticaria: It is a cutaneous condition characterized by erythema and wheal as a result of increased vascular permeability. Chronic urticaria > 6 weeks.
- Usually the lesions of idiopathic urticaria will resolve within minutes to a few hours in opposite to lesions developed in patients with urticarial vasculitis that will persist for > 24twenty-four hours and leaving depigmented mark.
- Urticarial vasculitis (UV) is defined as *chronic urticaria* usually for > six months and *leukocytoclastic vasculitis* in skin biopsy.
- UV is a rare disorder with an incidence about 0.5/100,000 persons, and HUVS occurs only in 1–2 percent and most of affected individuals are middle-aged women.

##There are three distinct subtypes in urticarial vasculitis spectrum (UV):

(A)Normocomplementemic Urticarial Vasculitis (NUV): This subtype is characterized by cutaneous lesions only with normal serum complements and has a benign course.

(B)Hypocomplementemic Urticarial Vasculitis(HUV): This subtype has a feature of cutaneous lesions only associated with low serum complements.

(C)Hypocomplementemic Urticarial Vasculitis Syndrome (HUVS): This subtype is considered the most severe form. Beside cutaneous lesions, the patients will have some systemic symptoms (eyes, kidneys, etc.).

★Pathogenesis:

- The etiology behind occurrence of HUVS is not well defined. However, IgG antibodies formation (mostly idiopathic or could be related to drug or infection or underlying

autoimmune disorders) against collagen, similar regions of C1q will enhance immune complex deposition and leads to complements activation.
- The activation of complements cascade will induce vascular inflammation in addition to immune complex deposition. As a result of that, vascular permeability will increase with mast cells degranulation leading to vasculitis and urticaria or angioedema.
- This pathological mechanism derived from (TYPE III) hypersensitivity reaction in which immune complex phenomenon is the dominant inducer for disease.
- Anti-C1q antibodies have been detected in pulmonary structure among patients with HUVS, raising the likelihood of pulmonary disease (COPD) in those patients as anti-C1q antibodies can cross with pulmonary surfactant.

★★Difference between urticaria and urticarial vasculitis:

Urticarial Vasculitis	Urticaria	Features
Burning pain	No	*Pain*
Yes	Yes	*Itching*
> twenty-four hours	Less than three hours	*Duration*
Hyperpigmentation	Complete	Resolution

> **★★Some atypical presentations of urticarial vasculitis (UV):**
>
> ^*AHA*: Arthritis, hives, and angioedema
>
> ^*Schnitzler's syndrome*: It is a rare autoinflammatory syndrome characterized by recurrent fever, nonpruritic urticaria, bony pain due to hyperostosis, and monoclonal gammopathy *IgM*.

★Clinical Assessment:

- By History:

CLINICAL NOTES IN VASCULITIC DISEASES

- Ask about history of urticaria (hives) associated with burning pain or angioedema.
- Ask about the duration of these cutaneous lesions (> twenty-four hours). Does this lesion leave any hyperpigmentation?
- Any history of joints pain or swelling or stiffness.
- History of recurrent fever or bony pain.
- Any features of eye pain and redness.
- Any history of nervous system involvement like headache, cranial, or peripheral nerves injury.
- Any history suggestive for chronic cough or SOB (COPD)?
- History of any GI manifestations like abdominal pain, nausea and vomiting, and diarrhea.
- Any history of hematuria or frothy urine?
- Ask about any symptoms of *lupus* (SLE) or Sjogren's syndrome (SS).
- History about recent drug use or recent infections.

-By Examination:

- Check the vitals (BP >>> HTN may point toward renal involvement).
- Check for any urticarial lesions and hyperpigmented areas.
- Do full neurological examination, *including full eye examination by ophthalmologist.*
- Rule out any synovitis!
- Examination for cardiovascular, pulmonary, and GI systems.

**Clinical manifestations of (HUVS):*

Skin	100%	Urticarial lesions or angioedema
Joints	70%	Arthralgia or arthritis
Kidneys	50%	Proteinuria, hematuria, RPGN
Gastrointestinal Tract	30%	Abdominal pain, nausea and vomiting, diarrhea or ascites
Lungs	20%	SOB or cough (COPD)
Eyes	10%	Episcleritis, uveitis, and conjunctivitis

Schwartz's Criteria (1982) for diagnosis of HUVS:

^^Major Criteria:

- Chronic urticaria of > six months
- Hypocomplementemia

^^Minor Criteria:

- Leukocytoclastic vasculitis in skin biopsy
- Arthralgia or arthritis
- Ocular inflammation
- Glomerular disease
- Abdominal pain
- Positive anti-C1q antibodies

====> All major criteria should be met, and more than or equal to two of minor criteria to define patients with HUVS.

====>*To diagnose HUVS, all other diseases should be excluded*–Mixed cryoglobulinemic vasculitis

- High level of anti-ds-DNA antibodies (SLE), and
- Decreased C1 esterase inhibitor level.

*Investigations:

>>>Basic labs:

- CBC with differentials: R/O leucopenia or thrombocytopenia associated with (SLE).
- Renal and hepatic profiles: acute kidney injury or rise in LFTs associated with cryoglobulins.

- Urinalysis or twenty-four-hour urine protein collection: hematuria or proteinuria to decide about systemic involvement in HUVS.
- ESR and CRP: elevated among patients with HUVS.
- Thyroid function test: TSH or FT4. Hypothyroidism can cause chronic urticaria.
- ANA and anti-dsDNA antibodies: R/O underlying hidden SLE.
- Anti-C1q antibodies: Positive result seen in > 90 percent among patients with (HUVS).
- Complements (C3/C4): can be normal or low among patients with UV. C1q, C3, or C4 complements are markedly declined among patients with HUVS.
- ANCA an cryoglobulins level should be requested.
- Hepatitis B, hepatitis C, and HIV serology: to be ordered, as viral infections by these microbes can cause urticaria.

>>>Basic imaging:

- Renal ultrasound: for assessment before renal biopsy if the patient has abnormal urinalysis.
- Abdominal ultrasound: to assess for hepatosplenomegaly.
- HRCT chest: for assessment of COPD if the patient is complaining of respiratory symptoms; otherwise, chest X-Ray (CXR) will be reasonable.
- Echocardiogram: R/O vegetations and atrial myxoma.

**Pathological assessment:* The site of biopsy: skin versus kidney if urinalysis is abnormal.

-*Skin:* Dermal perivascular inflammatory cells infiltrate mainly neutrophils with leukocytoclasia. You can assess for deposition of C1q in endothelium.

-*Kidney:* Immune complex-mediated GN (MPGN has been reported among HUVS).

*Simplified approach for diagnosis of patients with urticarial vasculitis (UV):

- You have to ask the patients about these urticarial lesion: acute or chronic, and when these lesions disappear. Do they leave any hyperpigmentation? Are they associated with pain or not?

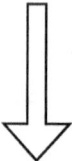

- If urticarial lesions are chronic, disappear in > twenty-four hours, associated with hyperpigmentation, and there is burning pain, most likely UV. At this point, we have to ask the patients about systemic symptoms of HUVS and symptoms of SLE, or any recent medications' usage or infections' risk factors, such as viral hepatitis.

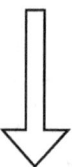

- After that, you have to request for labs to R/O mixed cryoglobulinemic vasculitis or underlying SLE. Also to identify which subtype of UV we are dealing with—NUV vs. HUV vs. HUVS? If HUVS is the diagnosis, try to recognize what are the major organs involved by disease to decide about your management plan.

*Differential diagnosis in case with urticarial vasculitis (UV):

- *Systemic Lupus Erythematosus (SLE):* It's hard to tell is it pure(SLE) or SLE occurs concomitantly with (HUVS). *When SLE patients present with uveitis, check anti-C1q antibodies.*
- *Mixed Cryoglobulinemic Vasculitis*
- *Familial autoinflammatory syndrome* like:

CLINICAL NOTES IN VASCULITIC DISEASES

- ∧ Cryopyrinopathies: Muckle-Wells syndrome characterized by defect in NLRP-3 gene with history of intermittent fever, joints pain, urticaria, and deafness.
- ∧ Schnitzler's syndrome: IgM gammopathy, fever, and hyperostosis.

  - *Congenital complement deficiency disorder:* History of recurrent infections.
  - *C1 esterase inhibitor deficiency:* History of recurrent angioedema.

*Management:

- The decision about treatment of UV is based mainly on manifestations.
- The treatment of cutaneous manifestations consists of oral antihistamine (H1-receptor antagonist = hydroxyzine) 25 mg PO q for eight hours, low-dose prednsiolone (0.3mg/kg/day), and try to taper the dose over four to six weeks.
- In case of refractory urticarial vasculitis or relapsing lesions upon tapering the course of steroid, additional immunosuppressive therapies should be considered, like MTX, azathioprine *2mg/kg*, MMF *1–2g/day*, cyclosporine, and cyclophosphamide.
- If the patient has HUVS with systemic organ manifestations like glomerulonephritis, steroid in high dose, cyclophosphamide, and other steroid sparing agents can be used after induction of remission.
- Rituximab (RTX) can be used in some cases; refractory to traditional immunosuppressive therapies as per case reports.

*Monitoring:

- Arrange the patients for regular follow-up to assess for cutaneous symptoms (Dermatology collaboration is paramount!).
- Ask about symptoms suggestive of major organs involvement like kidneys or lungs.
- Try to taper steroid as soon as possible to reduce the risk of steroid side effects.

===

*Anti-neutrophilic cytoplasmic antibody (ANCA)-associated vasculitis:

*Introduction:

- ANCA-associated vasculitis: Necrotizing vasculitis affecting small-sized blood vessels and characterized by presence of ANCA antibodies which directed either against *proteinase 3 PR-3* or *myeloperoxidase MPO*.
- ANCA-associated vasculitis group includes three major subtypes: granulomatosis with polyangiitis (GPA), microscopic polyangiitis (MPA), and eosinophilic granulomatosis with polyangiitis (EGPA).
- ANCA-associated vasculitis group: It is a rare disease with annual incidence about twenty per million population in Europe and North America.
- ANCA-associated vasculitis group tends to occur mostly equal between genders, with increasing in occurrence as the age progresses in the sixth decade of life.
- The most affected organs seen among patients diagnosed with ANCA-associated vasculitis are kidneys, lungs, upper respiratory tract, and nervous system.

**Subtypes of ANCA-associated vasculitis:

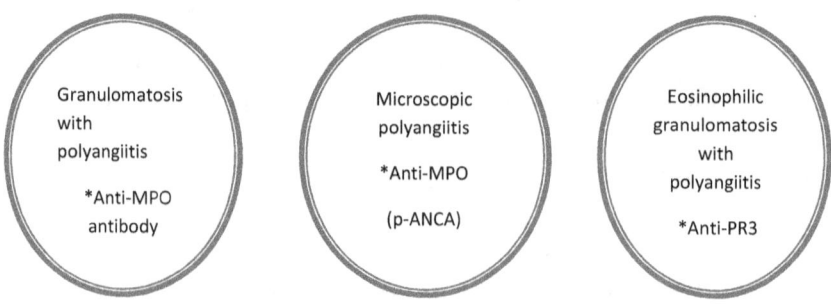

*Pathogenesis of ANCA-associated vasculitis:

- PR3 and MPO are cytoplasmic enzymes; *proteins* present mainly in granules of neutrophils and monocytes. These enzymes have antibacterial effect.

- Why antibodies develop against these cytoplasmic enzymes present in inflammatory cells? It's not clear. However, once neutrophils been activated by infectious microbe or having defect in apoptosis, prolonged stimulation of immune system by prolonged neutrophilic exposure or cross reactivity between these enzymes and microbial antigens may stimulate formation of (IgG) antibodies against these enzymes (ANCA antibodies).
- But the major question is why neutrophils attract to the endothelial layers of small blood vessels and producing symptoms of vasculitis. The answer is arising from when there is a microbial antigen or inflammatory cytokines like TNF-a, IL-1, lipopolysaccharide, or complement activation, such as C5a as a sequela of antigenic foreign stimulation. Neutrophils will be activated and cytoplasmic enzymes will be expressed on the surface of neutrophils.
- As a result of this process, antibodies released against these enzymes, and neutrophils will be more activated and causing increased expression of adhesion molecules, and neutrophilic degranulation will cause release of reactive oxygen species (ROS) with neutrophilic extracellular traps (NETosis) that lead to vascular endothelial injury. To promote more damage, chemokines and neutrophilic enzymes in the blood vessels will enhance the recruitment of T-cells.
- The importance of complement pathway in magnifying vascular inflammation among patients with ANCA-associated vasculitis has been identified, although affected individuals don't have any immune deposit. Binding of C5a to C5a receptor on neutrophilic surface will promote more neutrophilic activation with more C3 deposition (low C3). Hence, low C3 is associated with bad outcome.
- Finally, familial cases of ANCA-associated vasculitis have been reported with genetic defect in PRTN3 related to proteinase 3 enzyme and other genetic polymorphism is noted.

Granulomatosis with Polyangiitis (GPA):

- GPA is a necrotizing granulomatous inflammation affecting mainly upper and lower respiratory tracts and kidneys.
- It is commonly occurring between fifth to seventh decades of life.

^^*Manifestations of (GPA):*

- Upper and lower respiratory tracts involved in about 70–100 percent, otological involvement is seen among 35 percent, while kidneys are injured in about 50–80 percent.

> Upper respiratory tract manifestations: recurrent nasal discharge, epistaxis, nasal crusting and ulceration, depressed nasal bridge, and sinusitis with nasal fullness.
> Laryngeal and tracheal stenosis: hoarseness, stridor, and shortness of breath with subglottic stenosis is seen in 6–23 percent.
> Otological manifestations: SNHL, serous otitis media, chronic otitis media with mastoiditis, and inner ear symptoms (vertigo) due to immune complex deposition in the cochlear vessels.
> Lungs manifestations: Cough and shortness of breath, which could be related to fixed pulmonary infiltrate, or nodule or pulmonary cavitations. Also, the patients can present with hemoptysis due to capillaritis causing pulmonary hemorrhage.
> Oral cavity manifestations: painful or painless oral ulcer not involving hard palate with gingival hyperplasia and possibility of strawberry-like oral mucosa.
> Skin manifestations: purpura, skin ulcers, digital infarct.
> Eye manifestations: episcleritis, scleritis, conjunctivitis, retinal vasculitis, and hemorrhage and proptosis due to retro-orbital pseudotumor.
> Articular manifestations: arthritis, either erosive or not erosive.
> Central and peripheral nervous systems manifestations: headache, seizure, CVA, cranial neuropathies (facial nerve palsy), pachymeningitis, pituitary gland, spinal cord lesions, sensory or motor polyneuropathy, or mononeuritis multiplex.
> Kidneys manifestations: hematuria, frothy urine (proteinuria), or severe AKI happened acutely.
> Cardiovascular manifestations: cardiomyopathy due to occlusive small vessels disease, valvulitis, pericarditis, and pericardial effusion.
> Gastrointestinal manifestations: peritonitis, mesenteric ischemia (acute abdomen).

CLINICAL NOTES IN VASCULITIC DISEASES

> Genitourinary tract manifestations: GPA can manifest with urethritis, epididymo-orchitis, cystitis, penile necrosis, and ureteric obstruction by mass.
> Constitutional symptoms: fever, myalgia, malaise, arthralgia, weight loss, and anorexia. (Constitutional symptoms are commonly noticed among patients with GPA.)

#Be careful! Patients with GPA can present with granulomatous mass in the brain, eye, retroperitoneal cavity, and kidney, etc. *(R/O malignancy first!)*

- Patients diagnosed with GPA are divided into two major groups:
* Limited GPA: only respiratory tract (like nasal symptoms) involved.
* Diffuse GPA: upper respiratory tract and lungs (including cavitations) and kidneys involved. Any other major organs affected considered diffuse group.

>>*Ten percent of patients with limited disease will switch into diffuse disease.*

**ACR classification criteria for GPA: The presence of more than or equal to two of these criteria is considered significant *Se=88 percent and Spe=92 percent.*

1- Nasal or oral inflammation: Painful or painless oral ulcers or purulent or bloody nasal discharge.

2- Abnormal chest radiograph: Nodule or fixed infiltrate or cavitations.

3- Abnormal urinary sediment: Microscopic hematuria positive or negative red cells cast.

4- Granulomatous inflammation in tissue examination.

- ((75%)) of patients with GPA have positive C-ANCA while 20% have positive typical P-ANCA. Only 5% of patients are ANCA negative.

*Examination of patients with GPA disease:

1– Examine for vitals (Does the patient look unstable?). If with high BP and low oxygen saturation, *pulmonary hemorrhage,* >>> urgent referral to ICU.

2– Do upper and lower respiratory tracts examination: oral or nasal ulcers, nasal clots, or depressed nasal bridge, and you can ask the help from an *ENT* specialist to see if there is any perforated nasal septum, or do upper airway scope for subglottic stricture. Also, check for stridor and crepitations.
3– Eye examination by an ophthalmologist.
4– Central and peripheral nervous systems examination to see if there is any neuropathy, foot drop, or wrist drop.
5– MSK examination for synovitis.
6– Skin examination for purpura or skin ulcers; signs for illicit drugs injections.

*Investigations:

>>>Basic labs:

- CBC with differentials: to look for normochromic normocytic anemia or high platelets as acute phase reactant.
- Renal profile and urinalysis or twenty-four-hour urine protein collection: to assess for kidney function 7 presence of hemturia or proteinuria with active cast.
- Liver profile: to assess for any rise in transaminase due to mass effect or albumin level.
- Inflammatory markers: ESR and CRP may be elevated in diffuse disease. However, in some limited forms, it will not rise significantly. High procalcitonin will point toward infection.
- ANCA testing: By qualitative (IF) and by quantitative (ELISA) methods to increase sensitivity and specificity (c-ANCA among patients with GPA).
- Request for ANA, anti-ds-DNA antibodies, cryoglobulins, anti-GBM testing.
- Blood culture from two different sites. (Also, you can ask for rheumatoid factor if you are thinking about infective endocarditis.)
- Sputum culture is important.
- Viral serology: HIV, HBV, and HCV to be done.
- QuantiFERON-TB testing is extremely helpful to R/O tuberculosis.
- Urine toxicology: R/O cocaine-induced vasculitis.

- EMG/NCS: to check if there is any neuromyopathy.
- Bronchoscopy and BAL: hemorrhage *hemosiderin-laden macrophages* or culture.
- PFT and flow volume loop: R/O subglottic stricture.

>>>Basic imaging:

- CT nasal sinuses: sinus opacification.
- CT chest (HRCT): diffuse ground-glass opacities or bronchiectasis.
- Brain or spinal cord MRI: to assess for nervous system involvement if suggestive symptoms are present.
- Ultrasound liver and kidney: to see if there is any masses or to examine renal parenchyma before biopsy.
- Transthoracic echo: to exclude infective endocarditis (important differential diagnosis).

^^*Don't depend only on chest X-Ray (CXR) to rule out pulmonary involvement among patients with GPA as it's not sensitive modality and it can miss nodular changes!*

*Pathological assessment in GPA:

- Taking tissue sample from affected organs or granuloma is highly recommended.
- Tissue sample from upper respiratory tract: low diagnostic yield while open lung biopsy can show granulomatous or nongranulomatous lesion with pulmonary vasculitic lesions.
- Nerve and muscle biopsy: can show vasculitic lesion.
- Skin biopsy: will show leukocytoclastic vasculitis.
- Kidney biopsy: few or no immune complex deposit, crescentic necrotizing (Pauci-immune) glomerulonephritis. In some cases with ANCA-associated vasculitis, no glomerular lesions seen, but we should look for interstitium to recognize if there is interstitial nephritis due to vasa recta involvement or medullary angiitis. *(Granuloma is not seen in the kidneys.)*

*Differential diagnosis in case with GPA:

1– Other types of vasculitis: MPA/EGPA, PAN, CryoVas.
2– Anti-GBM disease (Goodpasture syndrome): No upper respiratory tract involvement and renal biopsy will show linear immune complex deposition.
3– Malignancy: NHL or NK/T-cell lymphoma can cause midline destructive lesion.
4– Sarcoidosis: Non-caseating granuloma with hilar lymphadenopathy.
5– Medications-induced: antithyroid drugs or cocaine that can induce hard palate destruction with positive c-ANCA and anti-HNE.
6– Infectious causes like: tuberculosis or *infective endocarditis*.

> **There is no clear diagnostic criteria for GPA, hence the diagnosis is usually dependent on clinical manifestations in combination with positive ANCA testing and histopathology! *Rule out vasculitis mimickers.*

*Microscopic Polyangiitis (MPA):

- It is a rare necrotizing vasculitic inflammation affecting mainly the kidneys, lungs, and nervous system.
- It is occurring commonly among patients in older age group in their sixth to eighth decade of life.
- There is *no* granuloma seen among patients with MPA. Eye and ENT symptoms are not frequently seen among patients with MPA.
- The diagnosis of MPA will base on clinical picture, biopsy, and labs (ANCA).

^^Manifestations of (MPA)

> Renal manifestations (80–100 percent): The patients can present with picture of *RPGN* or slowly progressive chronic kidney disease.
> Pulmonary manifestations (55–80 percent): Pulmonary hemorrhage is the most dominant clinical feature (cough,

SOB, and hemoptysis). ILD like *pulmonary fibrosis* can be a sequela of MPA.
> Cutaneous manifestations (30–60 percent): Palpable purpura is the most common cutaneous feature seen; however, nodule, livedo reticularis, and skin necrosis can be noticed.
> Neurological manifestations (37–72 percent): Mostly symptoms related to peripheral nerves, *mononeuritis multiplex and symmetrical polyneuropathy,* and central nervous system involvement occurs less frequently, like cerebral hemorrhage, infarction.
> Gastrointestinal manifestations (30–58 percent): abdominal pain is the most common symptom followed by GI bleeding.

*Examination of patients with MPA:

1-Check the vitals: assessment for BP, tachycardia, or hypoxemic patients due to pulmonary hemorrhage.

2-Check for central or peripheral nervous systems involvement: any focal deficit or sensory disturbance.

3-GI examination: any abdominal tenderness or signs of acute abdomen.

4-Cutaneous assessment for palpable purpura or skin ulcers.

*Investigations:

>>>Basic labs:

- CBC with differentials: to look for anemia. Anemia in the disease could be related to chronic kidney disease.
- Renal profile, urinalysis, and twenty-four-hour urine protein collection: Any rise in serum in creatinine, active urinary sediment, microscopic hematuria, or proteinuria.
- Liver function test: R/O any hepatic injury and to look for hypoalbuminemia.
- Viral serology for: HBV, HCV, and HIV to be requested.
- QuantiFERON-TB to be ordered.
- Blood cultures from two different sites: R/O bacteremia.
- Urine toxicology: in patients suspected to be a drug abuser.
- ANCA testing by IF and ELISA is important: 60 percent of patients with MPA have positive typical positive p-ANCA, with 30 percent having positive c-ANCA. Only 10 percent of the patients with MPA have negative ANCA testing.

- ANA, anti-dsDNA antibodies, anti-GBM, and cryoglobulins: R/O any other subtype of vasculitis or any autoimmune CTD.
- EMG/NCS: to assess for neuropathy and muscle involvement.
- Bronchoscopy and BAL: to check if there is any pulmonary hemorrhage or infection by sending culture from BAL.
- PFT: restrictive pattern due to pulmonary fibrosis.

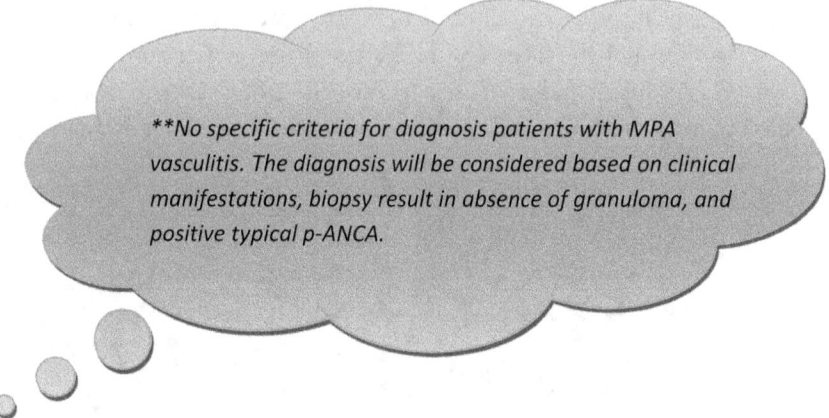

**No specific criteria for diagnosis patients with MPA vasculitis. The diagnosis will be considered based on clinical manifestations, biopsy result in absence of granuloma, and positive typical p-ANCA.

>>>Basic imaging:

- CT chest: to recognize any ground-glass opacities to R/O pulmonary hemorrhage or chronic interstitial infiltrate (UIP pattern).
- Transthoracic echocardiography: R/O vegetations.
- Brain MRI if the patient has any neurological symptoms: you can see either hemorrhage or infarct.
- CT abdomen and pelvis if the patient developed any GI manifestations: R/O mesenteric ischemia.
- Ultrasound kidneys: to assess renal parenchyma before biopsy.

*Pathological assessment in MPA:

- Tissue sample is crucial in reaching the diagnosis among patients with ANCA-associated vasculitis.
- MPA is characterized by necrotizing vasculitic lesions in renal and open surgical lung biopsy specimens.

CLINICAL NOTES IN VASCULITIC DISEASES

- Kidneys, lungs, and nerves—all of them can be a suitable site for biopsy once these organs have been affected.
- Renal biopsy will show: necrotizing crescentic glomerulonephritis (Pauci-immune) with possibility to see focal thrombosis of glomerular capillaries with fibrinoid necrosis.
- Open lung biopsy will show: vasculitic lesions *capillaritis*.
- Skin Biopsy: leukocytoclastic vasculitis (not specific).

---

*Differential diagnosis in case with MPA:

1-Other subtype of ANCA-associated vasculitis: like GPA with absence of granuloma is critical in MPA.

2-Other vasculitis: like CryoVas, anti-GBM disease, or drug-induced ANCA vasculitis.

3-Other CTD like: SLE.

4-Infectious cause like: endocarditis (positive typical p-ANCA 5 percent).

5-Other disease causing positive atypical p-ANCA like: cystic fibrosis or primary sclerosing cholangitis.

---

*Eosinophilic granulomatosis with polyangiitis (EGPA):

- It is an eosinophilic-rich necrotizing granulomatous vasculitis involving mainly upper and lower respiratory tracts.
- It is characterized mainly by late-onset asthma with peripheral eosinophilia.
- EGPA mainly occurs in individuals between age forty to sixty years.
- ANCA positivity is seen among 40 percent of patients diagnosed with EGPA.

Pathogenesis of EGPA

^ The pathogenic pathway responsible for development of EGPA manifestation is complicated. It reflects the interaction between genetic background like HLA-DRB1*04, HLA-DRB1*07, and HLA-DRB4 that cause abnormal T-cells response and environmental triggers like infections, drugs, and vaccinations.

^ As a result of this complicated interaction, Th-2 cells will be stimulated via IL-4, IL-5, and IL-13.

^ Additionally, the role of eosinophils in pathogenesis of EGPA is not well known. However, its stimulation and attraction toward the site of inflammation by chemokine (eotaxin-3) will positively enhance the function of T-cell by production of IL-25 by eosinophils.

∧ The implication of B cells in pathogenesis of EGPA is less recognized in comparison to T-cells. B cells play a role in production of ANCA antibodies against MPO, with increment in IgG4 level in the sera of the patients diagnosed with EGPA. The number of clinical manifestations correlate with the rise in IgG4 level.

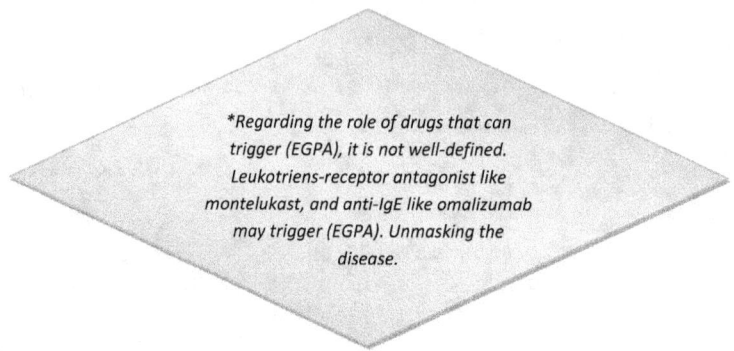

*Regarding the role of drugs that can trigger (EGPA), it is not well-defined. Leukotriens-receptor antagonist like montelukast, and anti-IgE like omalizumab may trigger (EGPA). Unmasking the disease.

★*There are three phases of (EGPA):*

#*First Phase: The prodromal (allergic) phase*: Started earlier at second to third decades of life, with history of asthma and allergic rhinosinusitis.

#*Second Phase: The eosinophilic phase:* Peripheral eosinophilia is dominant and infiltration of heart, lungs, and GI tract by eosinophils will occur.

#*Third Phase: The vasculitic phase:* The patients will have complained from vasculitic symptoms like purpura, neuropathy, and glomerulonephritis. Also, the patients at this phase will have constitutional symptoms more frequently.

★*Manifestations of EGPA:*

> Symptoms of asthma: noticed in about 95–100 percent and usually is developed in adulthood.

CLINICAL NOTES IN VASCULITIC DISEASES

> Symptoms of rhinosinusitis: 70–90 percent of patients with EGPA have symptoms of rhinosinusitis associated with nasal polyps in about 50 percent.
> Symptoms of lung involvement: SOB, cough, or hemoptysis with migratory lung infiltrate in the peripheral areas noticed ~ P38 percent, while pleural effusion is seen in 8.9 percent, and pulmonary hemorrhage is rarely seen among patients with EGPA in 4.2 percent.
> Cutaneous manifestations: seen in ~ 40 percent with purpura, necrotic skin lesions, livedo reticularis, or subcutaneous nodules.
> Symptoms of peripheral neuropathy: Almost 50 percent of patients with EGPA will have neuropathic features, while CNS manifestations are seen in ~ 5 percent.
> Cardiovascular manifestations: seen in about 27 percent in the form of cardiomyopathy *nonischemic*, pericarditis, valvulopathy, or intracardiac thrombus.
> Gastrointestinal manifestations: The patients with EGPA will develop GI complaint including urgent conditions like acute abdomen in about 23 percent.
> Kidneys manifestations: Kidney involvement is seen in 21 percent of patients diagnosed with EGPA and considered less common manifestation in opposite to GPA and MPA.
> Deep venous thrombosis: 7–10 percent of patients with EGPA have picture of DVT.
> Constitutional symptoms: Fever, myalgia, arthralgia, and weight loss seen in about 38–49 percent.

**In general, the manifestations documented among patients with EGPA are divided into two distinct groups:

-*Vasculitic manifestations (typical p-ANCA positive):* purpura, alveolar hemorrhage, glomerulonephritis, and neuropathy.

-*Eosinophilic manifestations (typical p-ANCA negative):* cardiac involvement and pulmonary infiltrate.

*(1990) ACR classification criteria for Churg-Strauss Syndrome (EGPA): (Four of six criteria should be met "Se.=85 percent and Spe.=99 percent.)

- Asthma,
- Eosinophilia (more than 10 percent of total WBC),
- Neuropathy,
- Non-fixed pulmonary infiltrate,
- Paranasal sinus abnormalities, and/or
- Extravascular eosinophils by biopsy.

*Lanham diagnostic criteria for diagnosis of EGPA:

All three criteria should be met for diagnosis:
- asthma,
- peripheral eosinophilia > 1500/mm3 or > 10 percent of total WBCS, and
- evidence of vasculitis in more than or equal to two organs.

*Examination of patients with EGPA:

1- Check the vitals. Tachycardia or tachypnea?

2- Does the patient have desaturation due to pulmonary hemorrhage?

3- Examination of respiratory and cardiovascular systems >>> Signs of heart failure or wheezing due to asthma?

4- Examine nasal cavity for any visible polyps or sinus tenderness.

5- GI examination for any acute abdomen.

6- Observe for any palpable rash!   7- Check for any neuropathy (wrist or foot drop).

*Investigations:

>>>Basic labs:

1– CBC with differentials: Eosinophilia in > 10 percent is found in all patients diagnosed with (EGPA).

2– Renal profile, urinalysis, twenty-four-hour urine protein collection: Increased creatinine, hematuria or proteinuria, or any abnormal sediments.

3– Hepatic profile: To assess hepatic function before prescribing any immunosuppressive medications.

4– ESR and CRP: are raised during active inflammation (non-specific).

5– Typical p-ANCA testing: The test is positive in about 40 percent, and negative result doesn't exclude the presence of EGPA.

6– Serum IgE level: The level of IgE is high among patients with EGPA.

7– Stool testing for ova and parasites: To exclude any helminthic or parasitic infections causing eosinophilia.

8– Eotaxin-3 (eosinophilic chemoattractant): Novel testing that measures the level of eotaxin-3 with high specificity and sensitivity for EGPA.

9– Hepatitis B and C serology: Before initiating any immunosuppressive medications.

10– HIV testing and QuantiFERON-TB: Are important to be requested.

11– Serum IgG-specific for aspergillus fumigates: Its positivity will increase the likelihood for ABPA.

12– Peripheral blood sample for flow cytometry: To rule out any hematological malignancies associated with eosinophilia.

13– Molecular testing for FIP1L1/PDGFR alpha mutation: This mutation is seen among patients with hypereosinophilic syndrome (HES) myeloproliferative variant.

14– Pulmonary function test (PFT): To help in identification of reversible airway obstruction, *asthma*.

15– Bronchoscopy and bronchoalveolar lavage (BAL): To determine any alveolar hemorrhage or to measure eosinophils in BAL, as a high count in the fluid is consistent with EGPA. Also, sending for microscopy and cultures from fluid is important.

16– Electromyography or nerve conduction study: To detect any neuropathy which could be helpful as a site for biopsy.

>>>Basic imaging:

1– Chest X-Ray (CXR): It may show pulmonary infiltrate or nodules.
2– CT chest: To assess for alveolar hemorrhage or migratory infiltrate.
3– CT abdomen and pelvis: In case of presence of GI symptoms to rule out acute abdomen!
4– Renal ultrasound: To examine renal parenchyma before biopsy if labs indicate nephropathy.
5– GI endoscopy: It is an important tool in case of GI involvement as it can visualize ulcers in small intestine like duodenum.
6– Echocardiography: To evaluate cardiac function for cardiomyopathy, pericardial effusion, and intracardiac thrombi.
7– Cardiac MRI: Abnormal gadolinium enhancement can give us an idea about cardiomyopathy.

*Pathological assessment in EGPA:

- Taking tissue sample from affected organs is an extremely important step to confirm the diagnosis of EGPA.
- Kidneys, sural nerve and muscle, skin and GI tract: All of them can be a site for biopsy.
- The finding in biopsy: necrotizing granulomatous vasculitis with extravascular eosinophilic deposition. (Kidney biopsy will not show granuloma formation!)

*Differential diagnosis in case with EGPA:

1-Other ANCA-associated vasculitides: Patients diagnosed with either *GPA* or *MPA* do not have eosinophilia and asthma (neuropathy more common in EGPA).

2-Hyepreosinophilic syndrome (HES): No asthma among patients with HES and not presenting with vasculitic symptoms like purpura. Molecular analysis for mutation is paramount.

3-Parasitic and helminthic infections: No asthma or vasculitic manifestations among those patients.

4-Allergic bronchopulmonary aspergillosis (ABPA): No vasculitic phenomenon, and requesting serum specific antibodies for aspergillosis and ordering sputum examination for hyphae are critical steps.

*Management of ANCA-associated vasculitis:

\>\>The management of each subtype will be discussed separately.

\>\>It is important to identify earlier if the patients need *ICU* care like intubation or urgent hemodialysis.

\>\>The management in this type of vasculitis involves two steps approach: induction phase (three to six months) to suppress the inflammatory process, and maintenance phase (twenty-four to forty-eight months) to prevent recurrence of the disease.

> *All these manifestations should be treated as diffuse GPA disease:
>
> A-Pulmonary nodules with cavitations \\ B- Deafness \\ C- Purpura with ulceration

#Management of GPA: *You can calculate BVAS score to assess activity as it is a comprehensive tool.*

- The management of GPA vasculitis is dependent on the burden of disease (limited vs. diffuse); induction phase followed by maintenance therapy.
- Multidisciplinary approach is important, including nephrology, pulmonology, and ICU teams.

**INDUCTION of REMISSION:

- Diffuse disease subset of GPA can be managed by high dose glucocorticoids with pulse dose ~ 15 mg/kg daily for three days, followed by 60 mg PO daily and the dose to be tapered over three to six months and either cyclophosphamide (CYC) or rituximab (RTX).
- Cyclophosphamide (CYC) ~ 2mg/kg/day can be used either in oral form or it can be given intravenously ~ 15mg/kg every two weeks for three doses, then 15mg/kg every three weeks for another three to four doses. NIH protocol can be used.
- CYCLOPS trial is unblinded controlled trial that randomized 149 patients with *GPA/MPA* to receive either daily or pulse

IV regimens of cyclophosphamide. The proportion of the patients achieving remission was same between two arms, and leucopenia was lower among patients on pulse IV regimen. However, the risk of relapse was lower among patients who received oral form over ~ four years due to high cumulative amount of cyclophosphamide.
- Rituximab (RTX) is another medication that can induce remission among patients diagnosed with *GPA/MPA*. The regimen can be weekly with the dose of ~ 375 mg/m2 weekly for four weeks, or two doses of 1 g separated by two weeks.
- RAVE trial: 197 patients diagnosed newly with *GPA/MPA*, or with relapsing pattern randomized to receive either RTX weekly form or CYC IV pulse form followed by azathioprine. Complete remission off glucocorticoids at six months was seen in 64 percent of patients who received RTX compared to 53 percent of patients on CYC. No significant difference was noticed between RTX or CYC in relapse rate and in the rates of adverse events (RTX non-inferior to CYC).
- EUVAS trial or RITUXVAS: 44 patients with severe renal involvement ANCA-associated vasculitis was randomized to receive either RTX weekly and two doses of IV cyclophosphamide, or IV cyclophosphamide over three to six months followed by azathioprine. Both groups attained remission at similar percentage (76 percent vs. 82 percent) with similar rate of adverse events.
- *Be Careful!* RAVE trial excluded patients presented with severe renal insufficiency (Creatinine > 354 mcmol/L or dialysis) and they avoided to include patients presented with alveolar hemorrhage requiring mechanical ventilation. As a result of that, in such two critical conditions, many experts advised to use cyclophosphamide IV or RTX weekly for four weeks and two doses of IV cyclophosphamide.
- Regarding the use of methotrexate (MTX) in induction of remission among patients diagnosed with GPA, there is one trial called NORAM trial that included one hundred patients mostly diagnosed with GPA, but those patients didn't have any organ-threatening manifestations randomized to receive either MTX or oral cyclophosphamide for twelve months. The remission rate at six months was almost equal in both arms. However, more

patients on MTX relapsed at eighteen months. Hence, MTX can be used as induction therapy in cases characterized with non-severe manifestations like sinus disease, etc.
- Interestingly, mycophenolate mofetil (MMF) has been discussed in different studies as a drug that can be used for induction of remission among patients with ANCA-associated vasculitis. The most important study is the MYCYC trial which included 140 patients diagnosed with *GPA/ MPA with renal involvement eGFR>15 ml/min/1.73m2* and were randomized to receive either MMF 2–3 g/day or IV cyclophosphamide. It had been shown that MMF is non-inferior to CYC in percentage of remission at six months. However, more patients on MMF relapsed, especially patients with positive anti-PR3 antibody. MMF can be considered as a line for induction of remission in addition to glucocorticoids among patients with positive anti-MPO antibody with mild to moderate renal impairment without severe manifestations.
- As complements play an important role in pathogenesis of ANCA-associated vasculitis, ADVOCATE trial tried to study the effect of avacopan, C5a receptor inhibitor, on remission at twenty-six weeks in comparison to prednisone. Avacopan was non-inferior to prednisolone at the level of remission rate. However, patients on avacopan achieved sustained remission at fifty-two weeks more in comparison to prednisone. All patients received either RTX or CYC.
- Plasma exchange (PLEX) has been used as a modality for treatment among patients presented with severe manifestations such as renal failure requiring dialysis or alveolar hemorrhage necessitating ventilatory support. PEXIVAS trial enrolled 704 patients with severe renal involvement *eGFR<50ml/ min/1.73m2,* or alveolar hemorrhage, or both, and those patients were randomized to receive either standard therapy and PLEX or standard therapy alone. No difference in the rate of ESRD or death was noticed between two arms, and this study didn't show any long-term benefit of PLEX. But there is an important point to identify what is the subtype of patients that may benefit from PLEX. Patients with ANCA positivity and positive anti-GBM antibody should prescribe for them PLEX therapy.

- Limited disease subset of GPA like sinonasal disease without bony erosion or can be managed in collaboration with expert otorhinolaryngologists to differentiate between active disease versus damage. Management by nasal irrigation with saline is important combined with high dose glucocorticoids ~ 1mg/kg PO once daily, tapered, and Methotrexate (MTX) ~ 15–25 mg PO once weekly and folic acid.
- There are some manifestations that may occur among patients with GPA and can cause substantial morbidity like subglottic stenosis, tracheobronchitis, and bronchial mass. The plan about treatment should be tailored with otorhinolaryngologists. Subglottic stenosis can be managed by intralesional steroid injection and dilation. Some reports indicate variable encouraging results and benefits about usage of steroid and MTX or RTX.
- Management of orbital inflammatory disease among patients with GPA is difficult as it carries a high risk for relapse. RTX is considered the favorite choice used to treat such condition in combination with steroid. *Ruling out lymphoma and IgG4-related disease is important!*

MAINTENANCE of REMISSION:

- After induction of remission by strong immunosuppressive agents (CYC vs. RTX), maintenance therapy is needed to prevent relapses.
- Azathioprine can be used as an agent for maintenance of remission as per CYCAZAREM trial that included 144 patients diagnosed with ANCA-associated vasculitis GPA/MPA who were randomized to receive either azathioprine or to continue on IV cyclophosphamide. The relapse rate over eighteen months was similar between two arms.
- Methotrexate (MTX) can be tried as an alternative for maintenance of remission among patients diagnosed with ANCA-associated vasculitis based on WEGENT trial. In this trial, they included 126 patients randomized to receive either azathioprine or methotrexate. Both arms have similar rates of relapse-free survival.

- Rituximab (RTX) is considered a valuable option for maintenance of remission among patients either newly diagnosed or with relapsing pattern based on:

  ^^ (MAINRITSAN 1 trial, which included 115 newly diagnosed or relapsing patients, randomized to receive either RTX 500 mg for two doses at two weeks apart, followed by 500 mg every six months for eighteen months, or Azathioprine for twenty-two months, and all patients received cyclophosphamide (CYC) for induction of remission. Azathioprine was associated with more severe relapses in comparison with (RTX) at *29 percent versus 5 percent.*

  ^^ RITAZAREM trial included 170 patients who have relapsing disease and were randomized to receive either RTX 1 g every four months or azathioprine, with all patients receiving rituximab (RTX) for induction of remission. Rituximab (RTX) was superior to azathioprine in preventing relapse with *13 percent versus 38 percent.*

- Mycophenolate mofetil (MMF) may be an option for maintenance therapy. However, its usage is associated with more relapse rate in comparison to azathioprine based on IMPROVE trial. It can be used for this purpose in patients whose disease is characterized by mild to moderate renal impairment with positive anti-MPO antibody.

Duration of maintenance therapy in ANCA-associated vasculitis:

#The optimal period for maintenance regimen among patients diagnosed with ANCA-associated vasculitis is debated.

#REMAIN trial: This trial showed azathioprine discontinuation at twenty-four months and was associated with more relapses in opposite to continuation of treatment for forty-eight months that was more sufficient to decrease relapse and improve renal survival.

#The duration varies between different reports; however, the most suitable duration is twenty-four months to forty-eight months (based on different studies).

> ****_Other supportive measures should be added during management of ANCA-associated vasculitis:_**
>
> 1. TMP-SMX: can be used to reduce the risk of PCP infection among patients receiving cyclophosphamide (CYC) and using steroid > 20 g/day for more than one month.
> 2. Nasal irrigation with saline in patients diagnosed with sinonasal disease.
> 3. Calcium and vitamin D prophylaxis to reduce the risk of osteoporosis.
> 4. Gastrointestinal prophylaxis by PPI to avoid occurrence of peptic ulcer disease.
> 5. Don't forget to screen for chronic infections before starting immunosuppressive drugs.
> 6. Vaccination against seasonal influenza, COVID-19 vaccine as per precautions, and pneumococcal vaccine.
> 7. Be careful about cardiovascular risk factors to avoid any impairment of any quality of life.

*Management of MPA:

- The treatment used for management of patients diagnosed with MPA is similar to medications used for management of GPA.
- Alveolar hemorrhage, renal involvement, central and peripheral nervous system involvement, and cardiac and GI involvement, all these organ-threatening conditions should be managed with induction phase followed by maintenance phase.
- Induction phase: High dose steroid and CYC versus RTX, followed by maintenance phase which includes azathioprine versus RTX for thirty-six to forty-eight months.
- The relapse rate among patients diagnosed with MPA with positive anti-MPO antibodies looks lower than patients diagnosed with GPA.
- Interstitial lung disease (ILD-UIP) is increasingly seen among patients with ANCA-associated vasculitis with positive

anti-MPO antibodies. If there are other manifestations of vasculitis present, the management will be the same as for other vasculitic symptoms. One-third of patients with ILD who have positive anti-MPO antibodies will develop vasculitic manifestations over time.

Kidney transplantation in ANCA-associated vasculitis:

> Acute glomerulonephritis (RPGN) that occurs in patients admitted with ANCA-associated vasculitis is responsible for irreversible organ damage.
> Patients labeled with ANCA-associated vasculitis who require dialysis due to (ESRD), renal transplantation is associated with decrease in all causes of death.
> Ideally, you should evaluate the patients who have *low eGFR < 20ml/min/1.73m2* without expected recovery for kidney function before dialysis.
> ANCA-associated vasculitis should be in remission for twelve months, and ANCA titer must be negative before transplantation.

Risk factors for relapse among patients diagnosed with ANCA-associated vasculitis:

1– Younger patients.
2– Positive anti-PR3 antibody (GPA).
3– Prior relapse. *If the patients had history of prior relapse and developed relapse late, is it better to keep the patients on maintenance therapy lifelong?*
4– Lung, upper respiratory tract, and heart involvement.
5– Preserved kidney function.
6– Short duration of maintenance immunosuppressive drugs.
7– Use MMF as a maintenance therapy.
8– B cells reconstitution post rituximab (RTX).
9– Increase in ANCA titers after remission. (Predictive for renal relapse.)

#Monitoring for patients diagnosed with ANCA-associated vasculitis:

- The physician should ask the patients to visit the clinic frequently, monthly, then every three months to assess for symptoms of BVAS, hypertension, renal function, and response to induction therapy.
- Request for urinalysis especially RBC cells, as proteinuria may persist for a while among those patients.
- You can request for ANCA titer as its increment may indicate relapse.
- B cell reconstitution may be an indicator for relapse (CD-19 > 0 and can be a tool used to determine the relapse is as per MAINRITSAN 2 trial on tailored group).
- Be careful about steroid side effects!
- Be careful about cyclophosphamide (CYC) and rituximab (RTX) side effects, like persistent non-glomerular hematuria in (CYC) group and hypogammaglobulinemia in (RTX) group!
- Screen the patients closely for cardiovascular risk factors!

*Management of EGPA: *Collaboration with a pulmonologist is paramount!"*

- The management of EGPA is dependent on calculation of five factors scoring system (FFS).
- FFS revised version 2011 includes the following: *"score 0–2 that means either the score will be zero, or FFS=1 when only one factor is present, or FFS=2 if two factors or more are present."*

1– Age is more than sixty-five years.
2– Cardiac involvement.
3– Kidney involvement with creatinine level > 150 mcmol/L.
4– Gastrointestinal involvement.
5– Absence of ENT manifestations. (The presence of these symptoms is associated with better prognosis.)

- Glucocorticoids is considered the cornerstone in EGPA management with a dose of *1 mg/kg/day,* tapered gradually to reach < 7.5 mg daily; steroid alone for management patients with *FFS=0.*

- Glucocorticoids and immunosuppressive therapies like cyclophosphamide (CYC) with a dose of *15 mg/kg* monthly for six to twelve months as an induction therapy. Steroid and immunosuppressive therapy for management patients with *FFS >= 1*.
- Also, other systemic manifestations such as central nervous system involvement, peripheral neuropathy, and alveolar hemorrhage, all of these symptoms should be treated with steroid and CYC as an induction therapy.
- In post-induction therapy, the patient should be continued on maintenance therapy like methotrexate (MTX = 15 mg once weekly and folic acid) or azathioprine at *2mg/kg/daily*. Maintenance therapy is to be continued for eighteen to twenty-four months.
- Rituximab (RTX) can be used as a line for treating the patients diagnosed with EGPA with refractory or relapsing pattern as per one retrospective study done in UK that collected sixty-nine patients. Those patients receive RTX as per RA protocol, then followed at six, twelve, eighteen, and twenty-four months. The improvement in BVAS was ~76 percent at six months and ~93 percent at twenty-four months. Also, there is reduction in steroid dose significantly. But we have to focus on relapse rate which was 54 percent at twenty-four months, and most relapses were related to asthma and ENT symptoms. Patients diagnosed with EGPA with positive anti-MPO antibody tend to have better response to RTX therapy and prolonged relapse-free survival.
- Mepolizumab with dose of *~ 300 mg subcutaneously monthly:* humanized monoclonal antibody against IL-5 that can decrease blood eosinophils count can be used for managing the patients with EGPA. Based on one double-blinded randomized placebo-controlled study (MIRRA trial), it showed that patients who received mepolizumab have more accrued weeks of remission at twenty-four weeks. Also, the remission occurs more among patients who received mepolizumab, and the dose of steroid decreased significantly in mepolizumab group at forty-eight to fifty-two weeks. Mepolizumab is considered a good option for patients with EGPA and predominantly active allergic symptoms.

- Other medications that can be tried in cases of EGPA: interferon-Alfa and IVIG, especially if the patients have debilitating neuropathic symptoms.
- The survival rates among patients diagnosed with EGPA at five and ten years from disease onset are 88–97 percent and 78–89 percent respectively.

---

*Monitoring and follow-up:

1- Try to arrange visits frequently during active disease to assess the patients for systemic and allergic symptoms (remission mean BVAS=0 with low dose of steroid except allergic symptoms).
2- Be careful about steroid side effects. Taper steroid gradually as the relapse increases during tapering.
3- Calcium, vitamin D prophylaxis, and vaccination are important!
4- TMP-SMX prophylaxis: Immunosuppressive agents can raise the risk of infection.
5- Predictors of relapse in EGPA disease: cutaneous involvement, lower eosinophils count at onset of disease, and positive ANCA titer.

##Drug-Induced ANCA-associated vasculitis (DI-AAV):

- It is a subtype of vasculitis that occurs mainly among young women and induced by some medications causing some manifestations occurred among patients with primary ANCA-associated vasculitis.
- This phenomenon is observed commonly among patients using anti-thyroid medications like propylthiouracil (PTU) and methimazole (MMI), with median prevalence ranges of 6–30 percent.
- The pathological or immunological aspects for occurrence of this phenomenon:

- The medications cause excessive activation of neutrophils that leads finally to increased production of neutrophilic extracellular traps (NETs).
- Abnormal degradation of NETs with increased formation leads to enhanced release of ANCA antibodies.
- Some medications can augment the release of B cells activating factor that stimulate B cells' response for production of autoantibodies.

   - The symptoms of DI-AAV are similar to the symptoms observed among patients with primary AAV. However, the course of disease tends to be milder in DI-AAV.
   - The target antigens of ANCA antibody will vary between different medications: MPO, lactoferrin, cathepsin G, and human neutrophilic elastase (anti-HNE in cocaine users).
   - The involvement of kidneys, lungs, nervous system, and high-grade fever tend to occur more frequently among patients with primary AAV.

> ^**Medications associated with DI-AAV:**
>
> A-Antithyroid medications like PTU and MMI (most common drugs causing DI-AVV, especially after eighteen months).
>
> B-DMARDs like sulfasalazine and anti-TNF-Alfa.
>
> c-Antimicrobial therapies: nitrofurantoin, TMP-SMX, minocycline, vancomycin, isoniazid, and rifampicin.
>
> D-Illicit drugs like: cocaine and levamisole.
>
> E-Miscellaneous drugs: clozapine, hydralazine, allopurinol, denosumab, and phenytoin.

★Investigations to be ordered in suspected cases with DI-AAV:

   - CBC with differentials: neutropenia can be seen among patients diagnosed with cocaine or levamisole-induced AAV.
   - Renal profile, urinalysis, twenty-four-hour urine protein collection: to see if there is any rise in urea or creatinine. If they were rising among patients with DI-AAV, they will not increase significantly.
   - Liver function test: liver enzymes may be elevated among patients using antithyroid medications or minocycline.
   - Positive ANA and positive anti-histone antibodies are found in some patients diagnosed with DI-AAV.
   - ANCA serology test: It could be typical p-ANCA or atypical.

- CRP: Its rise is not significant among patients diagnosed with DI-AAV.
- Biopsy from affected organs can be a target for investigations in group of patients diagnosed with organ-threatening conditions (RPGN, pulmonary hemorrhage).

*Management:

- The disease can present with either non-severe manifestations that can't threaten specific organ, or severe or organ-threatening manifestations.
- The immediate discontinuation of the offending drug is the mainstay therapy used for management of patients with DI-AAV in all cases.
- Non-severe manifestations like arthralgia and fever can be managed by stopping the drug alone. However, severe manifestations like RPGN and pulmonary hemorrhage should be managed with high dose steroid and strong immunosuppressive therapy.
- The duration of immunosuppressive therapy among patients with DI-AAV should be shorter than the duration for primary AAV, and maintenance agent may be not necessary to use it.
- You can follow the patients by asking about symptoms and (ANCA) titer.
- The prognosis of this phenomenon is generally better than the outcome among patients with primary AAV once the offending medication has stopped.

**Don't challenge the patients who had history of DI-AAV with the same offending medication or medication from same class, as the patients likely will develop DI-AAV again.*

- This group of vasculitis can affect any size and any type of blood vessels without specific predominance.

*Variable Vessels Vasculitis (VVV)

- This group (VVV) includes two important diseases:

- Behcet's Disease (BD), and
- Cogan's Syndrome (CS).

*Behcet's Disease (BD):

∧ Introduction:

- BD is a chronic, complicated subtype of vasculitis characterized by presence of recurrent oral or genital ulcerations. Other organs such as eyes, blood vessels, nervous system, and gastrointestinal system can be affected by (BD).
- It is a disease commonly occurring among patients from Middle East, the Mediterranean region, and eastern part of Asia such as Japan. The patients diagnosed with BD are from both genders, and the age of the patients is mainly between the second and third decades of life.

★Pathogenesis:

- The pathogenesis of BD is complex in which genetic (HLA-B51), geographical, and environmental or infectious triggers play a role in the development of variable presentations of BD.
- Innate immune system (dendritic cells or NK cells) and adaptive immune system with activation of both *Th1/Th17* can lead to increased production of different inflammatory cytokines: IL-17, IFN-gamma, and CXCL8.
- These inflammatory cytokines will stimulate neutrophils and cause neutrophilic hyper function with increased release of NETosis.
- The activated neutrophils will infiltrate perivascular tissues and cause organ damage.

★Clinical assessment:

> By History:

- Ask about history of recurrent oral ulcers which is considered the most important symptom documented among patients diagnosed with BD (three times per year). The ulcers are mainly minor (less than 1 cm) and can be single or multiple lesions that appear mainly in the tongue, gingival, and buccal

tissues. The lesions are painful, preventing the patients from eating, and take about two to four weeks to heal.
- Any history of genital ulcers: the second most common manifestations among patients with BD at *80–90 percent.* They are usually painful and leave scars after healing. Genital ulcers appear in males, mainly in the scrotum, shaft, and glans penis, while in females, they occur frequently in the labia. Perineum can be affected in both genders with BD. Don't forget to ask about sexual history, as STDs are considered one of the differentials.
- Cutaneous manifestations of BD at *28–80 percent:-* papulopustular or acneiform-like lesions present mainly in the face, trunk, or limbs. Other lesions, like follicular lesions, may appear. Erythema nodosum-like lesions manifest in about 15 percent and locate mainly over the lower limbs and characterized by pain and nodular texture. Also, pyoderma gangrenosum-like lesions can behave as large painful plaques.
- Are there any ocular symptoms like blurred vision, photophobia, hyperemia, floaters, and increased lacrimation? Ocular symptom occur in about *29–80 percent,* and tend to present as anterior or posterior or panuveitis. Ocular lesions are found more among male patients. Ocular symptoms represent poor prognosis among male patients. Retinal vasculitis may be found in patients diagnosed with BD.
- Any history of neurological manifestations (5–10 percent) like: headache, seizure, ataxia, hemiplegia, intracranial hypertension, confusion, and myelopathy. Cavernous sinus thrombosis may develop in patients diagnosed with BD). Peripheral nervous system-related symptoms are seen much less frequently in BD.
- Any articular symptoms (30–70 percent): non-erosive, nondeforming arthritis involving mainly knees, ankles, wrists, and elbow joints.
- History suggestive for any vascular events (up to 33 percent): Venous involvement is more common than arterial involvement. Venous attacks can be either superficial thrombophlebitis or picture of DVT that can affect any venous system. Arterial disease is observed either in form of thrombosis or aneurismal formation in arterial territories like

- pulmonary artery aneurysm, which is considered risky for the patients as the affected individuals are complaining usually of hemoptysis.
- Manifestations of gastrointestinal system involvement (0–45 percent): abdominal pain, diarrhea, vomiting, and hematochezia are dominant symptoms. *Ileocecal ulcers* are seen commonly in patients with BD with GI manifestations.
- Cardiac manifestations are seldom observed in patients with BD. However, there are many reported cases about myopericarditis and valvular lesions. Pericardial effusion +\- pleural effusion among immunosuppressed patients with BD, rule out *tuberculosis*.
- Features of epididymitis or orchitis may be noticed in BD: these features are not recurring frequently and tend to persist for a few days to weeks. Kidney involvement is not commonly reported in BD. Secondary amyloidosis can develop rarely among patients with BD having persistent active disease.

> By Examination:

- Do full neurological examination! Picture of meningeoencephalitis is prominent in individuals affected with BD.
- Ophthalmology referral is important in all patients diagnosed with BD.
- Check for any oral or genital ulcers with scarring. Also, you have to examine carefully for any cutaneous lesions, including cordlike lesions suggestive for superficial thrombophlebitis.
- Any features indicative of synovitis.
- Check for any signs of DVT in any limbs.
- Don't forget to do gastrointestinal examination, as *acute abdomen* may be a presentation in patient's diagnosed with BD. Additionally, examining the genitalia is important.

^^Pathergy testing:- subcutaneous needle prick "21-gauge" and waiting for 48 hours to detect any pustular formation (due to neutrophilic pathology and its positivity varies between different countries)

*International Criteria for Behcet's Disease (ICBD):

- Oral aphthosis = two points
- Genital aphthosis = two points
- Ocular lesions = two points
- Cutaneous lesions = one point
- Neurological manifestations = one point
- Vascular manifestations = one point
- Positive pathergy test (optional to be added) = one point

\>>If the patients collect more than or equal to four points, increase the probability of BD with sensitivity = 94 percent and specificity = 90.5 percent, with accuracy rate reaching up to 97 percent.

^^There is no specific test used to diagnose BD directly, and identifying patients with BD will depend on the criteria used for diagnosis and based on opinions from experts.

*Investigations:

\>>>Basic labs:

- CBC with differentials: to rule out any infectious causes.
- Renal profile or liver profile: before starting any therapy.
- ESR/CRP: could be elevated.
- HLA-B51: It is not a specific test and can be found even in normal population. HLA-B51 positivity is not present in any criteria used to diagnose BD. But if the test came back positive in patients diagnosed with BD, it may represent more severe disease phenotype.
- ANA, RF, and ANCA antibodies: should be negative.
- Hepatitis B and C and HIV serology: all should be requested.
- Serology for syphilis: genital ulcers can be caused by treponema pallidum but will not have other features of BD.
- QuantiFERON-TB: as we are living in endemic area in KSA, TB is considered an important differential diagnosis for a wide range of diseases.

>>>Basic imaging:

- CT pulmonary angiogram: in patients presenting with hemoptysis or before starting anticoagulation to rule out pulmonary artery aneurysm.
- Brain MRI, MRA, or MRV: among patients with BD who developed neurological symptoms. White matter hyper signal intensity lesions involving brain stem, cerebellum, and basal ganglia with picture of stroke-like lesions. Lumbar puncture will add a value for diagnosing *neuro-Behcet* with abnormal high WBC or protein and negative culture.
- Vascular angiogram or ultrasound with Doppler: Rule out any DVT or arterial aneurysms.
- Upper and lower (GI) endoscopy: Crohn's disease is a mimicker for BD, and the differentiation between these entities could be challenging. Patients with BD having GI symptoms will have single oval or rounded ulcers with focal distribution and the biopsy will not show granuloma.
- Echocardiogram: in case of suspicion of pericardial or myocardial involvement, although cardiac manifestations are not commonly present in BD.

*Pathological assessment: (It is not necessary for diagnosis.)

- From skin lesions: neutrophils-based inflammatory reaction.
- From CNS lesions: perivascular lymphocytic infiltrate with reactive astrocytes.
- From vascular tissues: increases in number of vasa vasorum infiltrated by lymphocytes and neutrophils.

**Simplified approach for diagnosis of patients with BD:

- If the patient has history of recurrent oral ulcers, you have to ask about other features of BD. Otherwise, patients can present with idiopathic recurrent oral aphthosis.

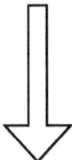

- Be careful! Genital ulcers may be related to venereal diseases like HSV, syphilis, and chancroid if they presented alone in context of typical history of sexual contact.

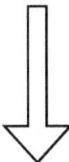

- In case of presence of neurological manifestations, exclude other differentials like infections or other autoimmune condition, like multiple sclerosis.

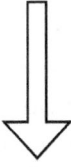

- Positive GI manifestations among patients with BD can be differentiated in difficult manner from IBD by doing biopsy, and always R/O celiac disease.

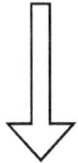

- Always, if you are suspecting patients to have BD, look for the patients from their whole aspects and ask yourself, Does this patient have other features present in ICBD? Don't be fooled by the presence of one manifestation and try to exclude other differentials mimicking BD.

★Differential diagnosis in case with BD:

1- Recurrent oral aphthosis alone could be an idiopathic disease. However, we have to rule out celiac disease, and malabsorption disorders like vitamin deficiency and herpes simplex infection.
2- Be careful! Exclude all causes of venereal diseases when the patient is presented with predominant genital ulcerations.
3- Crohn's disease is considered one of the important differentials among patients who developed GI manifestations.
4- Necrotizing vasculitis like (ANCA)-associated vasculitis.
5- In case of aneurysm or pseudoaneurysm, Takayasu's disease or PAN are considered important differentials.
6- MAGIC syndrome: a variant of BD characterized by mouth and genital ulcers with inflamed cartilage.
7- SLE is an important differential diagnosis in which the patients will develop cytopenia and renal involvement.

★Management:

> The choice of specific therapy among patients diagnosed with BD depends on manifestations of BD.
> Multidisciplinary approach is crucial for the right care.
> The management of each symptoms will be summarized alone.

^ *Management of mucocutaneous involvement:*

- Topical steroid (Trimacinolone 0.1 percent) three times a day over oral or genital ulcers.
- In case to prevent recurrence: colchicine should be tried first (0.6 mg PO BID).

- In case of refractory disease pattern: course of steroid can be initiated such as prednisolone 0.3 mg/kg/day (15–20 mg PO daily), tapered by 5 mg weekly.
- Additional steroid sparing agent can be added to help for complete discontinuation of steroid and to decrease recurrence such as azathioprine at 2.5 mg/kg/day.
- TNF inhibitors like infliximab, apremilast, thalidomide, or interferon alfa all can be tried in resistant cases.

^ *Management of eye involvement: (High morbidity)*

- Anterior uveitis can be managed by topical steroid eye drops. But among patients with BD who are male and of younger age, they tend to have poor prognosis.
- Hence, the initiation of strong immunosuppressive therapies since beginning is reasonably composed of high dose prednisolone at 1 mg/kg/day tapered over three months and azathioprine at 2.5 mg/kg daily.
- In case of severe disease judged by ophthalmologist: posterior, panuveitis, or retinal vasculitis, the treatment will involve high dose prednisolone and azathioprine, plus either cyclosporine at 2.5–5 mg/kg/day or infliximab.
- Tocilizumab use of TCZ 8mg/kg IV monthly has been reported among patients with BD who have features of eye or mucosal diseases, good result was seen in some cases.
- Rituximab (RTX) in *RA protocol* tried in some cases with mucocutaneous, eye disease and showed improvement in these symptoms (+\- MTX for eye disease).

^ *Management of gastrointestinal disease: (High mortality)*

- Patients diagnosed with BD with some GI manifestations, the diagnosis should be confirmed and we have to exclude: NSAIDs-induced gastrointestinal ulcer versus TB versus IBD.
- In case of acute abdomen, surgical team involvement since beginning is paramount in addition to immunosuppressive therapies.
- High dose prednisolone at 1 mg/kg/day and azathioprine at 2.5 mg/kg/day or 5-ASA.

- In case of resistant disease, TNF inhibitors, interferon alfa, thalidomide, or all of them can be tried when previous measures have failed.

∧ <u>**Management of vascular events (Angio-Behcet): (High mortality)**</u>

#The most important pathophysiological mechanism responsible for occurrence of thrombotic events is persistent vascular inflammation with increased level of reactive oxygen species that will perpetuate thrombus formation.

#The main therapy among patients with BD presented with thrombosis: high dose steroid and immunosuppressive agents.

#The addition of anticoagulation to immunosuppressive therapies should be done after weighing the risks and benefits, as anticoagulation drugs will not add any value in decreasing the risk of recurrence.

#If the decision about use of anticoagulants has been taken, you have to exclude vascular aneurysms to avoid occurrence of massive bleeding.

>>Venous thrombotic events (deep or superficial) in typical sites should be treated with: high dose steroidazathioprine, cyclosporine-A, adalimumab, or cyclophosphamide, +\- anticoagulation

>>Vena cava thrombosis should be treated with: high dose steroid and immunosuppressive therapies (CYC), +\- anticoagulation

>>Budd-Chiari syndrome should be treated with: high dose steroid and immunosuppressive drugs (CYC or TNFi).

>>Intracardiac thrombus should be treated with: high dose steroid, immunosuppressive agents (azathioprine or CYC), and anticoagulation. Triple therapy in intracardiac thrombi will lead to complete resolution in 78 percent of cases.

>>Central nervous system venous thrombosis (CNSVT) should be treated with: high dose steroid, immunosuppressive therapies

(azathioprine), and anticoagulation can be added. Combination therapy accounted for remission in about 85 percent.

\>\>Pulmonary artery involvement should be treated with: pulse steroid for three to five days, followed by a high dose steroid and cyclophosphamide (CYC). When pulmonary artery aneurysms and deep venous thrombosis are found, this is called (Hughes-Stovin syndrome). In case of refractory disease pattern, infliximab will be a good option.

\>\>Presence of pseudoaneurysms should be treated mainly by surgery preceded by steroid and azathioprine. Post-surgery, you can start a course of steroid and (CYC).

*Management of neurological involvement: (High mortality)

- Neurological involvement can either be parenchymal, involving mainly brain stem, basal ganglia, and spinal cord; non-parenchymal in form of sinus thrombosis; or aseptic meningitis.
- Treatment is composed of: pulse steroid therapy for three to five days, followed by high dose of steroid and CYC.
- In case of refractory disease pattern, we can try infliximab (IFX).
- Avoid use of cyclosporine-A in managing patients with BD having neurological symptoms, as cyclosporine-A can cause neurotoxicity.

*Management of articular disease:

- Colchicine should be an initial therapy in addition to low-dose steroid.
- Azathioprine and TNFi can be used in some resistant cases.

*Monitoring:

- BD is characterized by relapsing-remitting course, and we should follow the patients regularly and to ask them about any symptoms suggestive for major organs involvement, as the disease will be active in the first five to seven years.
- Be sure that patients with BD are taking the proper dose of azathioprine if this drug is being used (2.5 mg/kg/day) with

following the labs, as the dose less than the recommended will result in a high risk of flare.
- The duration of immunosuppressive therapies is ranging from two to five years, and the steroid sparing agent after this period can be tapered gradually.
- Multidisciplinary approach is important to help in optimizing the care provided to the patients.
- Try to decrease the dose of steroid to the lowest possible dose to decrease the risk of osteoporosis.
- Updated schedule for vaccination.

CLINICAL NOTES IN VASCULITIC DISEASES

*Cogan's Syndrome (CS):

*Introduction:-

- CS is a rare subtype of vasculitis characterized by the presence of ocular and audiovestibular symptoms.
- There is no gender predilection among patients diagnosed with CS, and most of the affected individuals are young in age (in the first three decades of their ages).
- It can attack different blood vasculature, and its manifestations can vary from less severe symptoms to large vessels involvement like *aortitis*.

*Pathogenesis:

- There is no clear mechanism that can explain the pathophysiology responsible for ocular and audiovestibular manifestations among patients with CS.
- However, the most suitable mechanism that can summarize the etiology is molecular mimicry with microbial antigens.
- Most of these microbes are reovirus type III that can cause symptoms of URTI, or chlamydia species being linked to pathogenesis of CS.
- Antibodies supposed to be released against these microbial antigens will cross-react with some corneal and inner ear extracts (Cogan's peptide). Moreover, these peptides tend to share some features with other antigens present on endothelial cells.
- As a result of release of these antibodies, the production of cytokines will be augmented and the inflammation will occur.

*Clinical assessment:

> By History: (Duration of symptoms is important.)

- You have to ask specifically about symptoms of inflammatory eye disease. The most common eye manifestations is non-syphilitic interstitial keratitis (IK) in which the patients can

have bilateral, irregular corneal infiltrate with redness and increased lacrimation.
- Don't forget to ask about other symptoms suggestive of eye disease (blurred vision, red eye, eye pain), and these could be a presentation for acute angle closure glaucoma, retinal vasculitis, retinal vein occlusion, conjunctivitis, optic neuritis, and scleritis.
- Also, taking deep history about audiovestibular manifestations is important, like tinnitus, hearing loss (unilateral versus bilateral), vertigo, and ataxia (Meniere's disease-like).
- Systemic manifestations are commonly present in *30–50 percent* among patients diagnosed with CS: fever, headache, arthralgia, arthritis, and myalgia.
- Cardiovascular involvement in CS at *10–28 percent* includes aortitis with aortic insufficiency that can manifest with heart failure.
- Patients with CS may also have some neurological symptoms (26 percent) like hemiparesis due to *CVA* or aphasia.
- Gastrointestinal symptoms can be seen among some patients diagnosed with CS (25 percent) like abdominal pain, diarrhea, and melena >>>? mesenteric arteritis.
- Moreover, cutaneous manifestations like purpura or urticaria may be found among patients with CS.
- Pulmonary manifestations like cough, dyspnea, and hemoptysis are sometimes present in patients with CS >>> interstitial pneumonitis.

> By Examination:

- Referral to ENT and ophthalmology teams is important to help in comprehensive evaluation for the patients.
- Cardiovascular examination: any murmurs, presence of HTN, orsigns of heart failure!
- Any signs for arthritis, purpura, lymphadenopathy, or splenomegaly?

> **There are two important variants of Cogan's syndrome (CS):
>
> (A) *Typical Variant*: non-syphilitic interstitial keratitis, audiovestibular symptoms, and the interval between these manifestation is less than two years.
>
> (B) *Atypical Variant*: other inflammatory ocular disorders and other audiovestibular symptoms, and the delay between these manifestations to appear is reaching > two years.

*Investigations: *(No specific diagnostic test!)*

>>Basic labs:

- CBC with differentials: Anemia, leukocytosis, and elevated platelet count may be seen among patients with CS.
- ESR: is rising among most of patients diagnosed with CS.
- Renal profile and liver profile: to check if there is any disturbance in renal and hepatic parameters; could by disease or to point to other pathology.
- Urinalysis and twenty-four-hour urine protein collection: sterile pyuria might be noticed in CS.
- ANCA level: may be positive in some patients diagnosed with CS, and can have elements of both diseases, especially ANCA-related GN.
- Hepatitis B and C, and HIV serology.
- QuantiFERON-TB before starting any treatment.
- Serology for syphilis is mandatory to be requested, as *syphilis* may cause all such manifestations.
- Some experts request anti-heat shock protein antibody (hsp70) in patients affected with CS and tends to be positive in 45–50 percent.

>>Basic imaging:

- MRA aorta: to help in early recognition of large vessels inflammation like aortitis.

- PET-CT scan: is very useful in identifying the extent of disease by assessing large vessels involvement.
- MRI/MRA of inner ear: mostly will be normal. However, some patients may have abnormal labyrinthine hyper signal intensity related to inflammation.
- MRI/MRA brain: to exclude any cerebellopontine angle tumor that can behave with similar audiovestibular symptoms.
- CT chest in case of suspicion of pulmonary hemorrhage or any other respiratory symptoms.
- Transthoracic echo: to evaluate cardiac function. Is there any valve abnormality like aortic insufficiency (AI)?
- Upper and lower GI endoscopy: in case of positive (GI) symptoms; can identify ulcerative lesions.
- <u>No specific site can be biopsied to give us the final diagnosis of CS.</u>

*Simplified approach for diagnosis of patients with CS:

\>\>\>Diagnosis of CS is dependent on the clinical picture of the patients.

\>\>\>Presence of sensorineural hearing loss and inflammatory ocular disease (IK) and all infectious or other inflammatory causes have been ruled out (mandatory elements in diagnosis), this is likely CS.

\>\>\>There are other prevalent additional symptoms in CS like: vertigo, ataxia, dizziness, tinnitus, fever, and weight loss.

\>\>\>Additionally, rising in inflammatory markers can add diagnostic value in proper clinical scenario.

*Differential diagnosis in case with CS:

- Infectious causes like *syphilis*.
- Other vasculitic syndromes like: Takayasu's arteritis (TA), granulomatosis polyangiitis (GPA), and Behcet's disease (BD).
- Sarcoidosis is an important differential especially among patients with dominant chest symptoms.
- Some autoimmune inflammatory condition that can present with ocular and audiovestibular symptoms like:

^^*Vogt-Koyanagi-Harada syndrome* or presence of uveitis, hearing loss, alopecia, and vitiligo without strong presence of vestibular symptoms; can be complicated with serous otitis media and retinal detachment.

^^*Susac's syndrome* or vasculopathy that involves retinal, cochlear, and cerebral vasculatures. The patients will manifest loss of visual acuity and hearing loss with vascular disease around corpus callosum in brain (MRI).

*Management:

- Multidisciplinary approach is extremely important in patients with CS.
- It is better to initiate glucocorticoids therapy as soon as the symptoms start to appear as the response to therapy will be enhanced if the inflammation is in its early phase, especially hearing defect.
- The cornerstone therapy in patients with CS is: high dose glucocorticoids at 1 mg/kg daily, tapered after two to three weeks when improvement is noticed till finishing the whole course within two-six months. Some reports indicate that IV glucocorticoids therapy can lead to significant improvement in hearing.
- Steroid sparing agents can be added like: methotrexate (MTX), azathioprine, mycophenolate mofetil (MMF), cyclophosphamide (CYC), anti-TNF-alfa (TNFi), rituximab (RTX 500 mg weekly for four doses), and cyclosporine-A. These agents can be included in the plan of therapy to prevent relapse or to treat resistant cases and decrease the steroids' side effects.
- The most suitable approach to start the patients with CS on high-dose steroid and TNFi (mainly infliximab 3mg/kg), +\- MTX, or azathioprine.
- Referral to ENT surgery for cochlear implantation is important as there are many patients who will not experience a good response in hearing to immunosuppressive therapies. So cochlear implant is a valuable option in such cases to preserve the quality of lives of these patients.

*Monitoring:

- In the beginning, try to arrange close follow-up after *three to four weeks* to determine the response to therapy, especially hearing impairment.
- Be cautious about steroid side effects (vaccination, osteoporosis, or prophylaxis)!
- Each visit, talk to the patients about symptoms of heart failure or GI symptoms to discover major organs involvement earlier.

-Poor prognostic factors in CS:

^^cardiac involvement,
^^ presence of (GI) symptoms,
^^positive history of weight loss,
^^high ESR,
^^anemia, leukocytosis, and high count of platelets.

> *Isolated (single) Organ Vasculitis*

*Cutaneous leukocytoclastic vasculitis (cLCV):

*Introduction:

- Cutaneous vasculitis: This is a term used to describe inflammation of small vessels located in the dermis and subcutaneous tissues.
- Cutaneous vasculitis: It can present with isolated skin involvement or can occur as a result of systemic autoimmune disorders.
- Taking full history and doing comprehensive examination are extremely mandatory to reach the correct underlying process responsible for cLCV.
- Deep *punch* tissue biopsy is necessary to identify inflammatory cells and to send for immunofluroscence examination (IF).

*Pathogenesis:

- The pathogenic phenomenon responsible for cLCV is not well defined. However, a complex interaction between the insult and immune system can explain such pathology.
- When triggers such as microbes, drugs, and malignant cells are present, the immune system will respond by releasing different antibodies that can form circulating immune complex particles.
- After immune complex particles have been deposited in the wall of blood vessels (post-capillaries), complement system will be activated.
- Once complements present at the site of injury, attraction of neutrophils and other inflammatory cells will occur.
- As a result of activation of neutrophils, the cells will degranulate and release nuclear dust.
- Additionally, activated neutrophils will produce cytokines and collagenases that induce vascular damage.

*Clinical assessment:

>>By History:

- Ask about purpura (site, onset, duration, and association with pain or not).
- Is there any history of bleeding tendency? (Bleeding diathesis can cause purpura-like.)
- Don't forget to ask about any other symptoms suggestive of different organs involvement (joints, respiratory symptoms, renal symptoms, etc.).
- Important question! History of recent drug use (especially antibiotics B-lactams).
- History of recent infections (bacterial, viral, TB)!
- Symptoms of other major autoimmune (CTDs) like SLE, pSS, dermatomyositis, and other subtypes of vasculitis.
- History of malignancies: solid and hematological tumors.
- Any symptoms of IBD?

>>By Examination:

- Observe for vitals (febrile or not, or hypertensive or not).
- Examine purpura (palpable or not?).
- Check if there are any features of synovitis.
- Respiratory and cardiovascular examinations are necessary.
- Signs for malignancies (check weight, lymph nodes enlargement, and hepatosplenomegaly).

*Investigations:

>>>Basic labs:

- CBC with differentials: look for infectious causes.
- Blood smear: any hematological malignancies >>> *plasma cells dyscrasias (PCD)!*
- Renal and hepatic profiles: extent of systemic disease or any exposure to toxins. (Remember, *send for urine toxicology!*)

- Urinalysis and twenty-four-hour urine protein collection: any active urinary sediment or proteinuria in case of systemic disease.
- Serum and urine protein electrophoresis: (PCD).
- Full septic screen: blood and urine culture ruling out bacterial sepsis.
- Hepatitis B and C, and HIV serologies: viral particles may cause cutaneous angiitis.
- QuantiFERON-TB to be ordered.
- Autoimmune profile: ANA, ENA group, ANCA level, complements level, and cryoglobulins level.

>>Basic imaging:

- Chest X-Ray: exclude hidden focus of infection.
- Other imaging modalities: based on the presentation of the patients.
- Echocardiography: Infective endocarditis is an infectious process that can behave with a picture very close to systemic vasculitis.
- Screen for malignancies if clinically indicated (family history, older age group, presence of constitutional symptoms, and absence of other explanations for these skin lesions).

Pathological assessment: *(Skin Biopsy!)*

- Neutrophilic nuclear materials (leukocytoclasia), and destruction of the wall, and extravasations of RBCs
- -Immunofluroscence staining is important. (Is there IgA deposit? >>> HSP)

DR. FAISAEL ALBALWI

*Simplified approach for diagnosis patients with (cLCV):-

^^A patient referred to your clinic because of palpable purpuric rash ?

⇩

^^You should ask yourself why these lesions developed.

Taking deep history and doing full examination is necessary.

⇩

^^Request complete work-up, including *skin biopsy.*

#If you can, review the biopsy with an expert pathologist!

⇩

^^The etiology will be mainly related to:

- ~Idiopathic (Primary) 30% – 70%
- ~Drug-related 8% – 36%
- ~Infections 9% – 36%
- ~Systemic autoimmune diseases 6% – 25% SLE, pSS, IBD, etc.
- ~All malignancies 2% – 8%

CLINICAL NOTES IN VASCULITIC DISEASES

> #*Important points you should pay your attention to while you are reading the report of the pathologist:*
>
> - *Not only neutrophils can infiltrate wall of the vessels.*
> - *When lymphocytes predominate, think about SLE, pSS, and some viral infections.*
> - *When granuloma is present, think about: GPA, sarcoidosis, Crohn's disease, and TB.*
> - *When IgA combined with IgM is seen in (IF) staining, think about: systemic causes, drugs related, or idiopathic.*

*Management:

- **The decision to treat patients diagnosed with cLCV is dependent on:**

    ~Is it isolated disorder or part of systemic disease?
    ~Is there any trigger like infections or drugs?

- *There are some conservative measures that can be used like rest, leg elevation, and compression stocking!*
- *Drugs can be used to treat cLCV:*

A- Prednisolone (0.5–1 mg/kg/day) tapered gradually over four to six weeks, especially when there are necrotic or ulcerative or blistering lesions found. A lower regimen up to 20mg/day can be used in case of simple purpuric rash.

B- Other medications that can be used in case of refractory or relapsing rash or chronic course:

   **Azathioprine = 2 mg/kg/day
   **Colchicine = 0.6 mg PO BID   *Colchicine and dapsone are used when neutrophilic lesions are present.*
   **Dapsone = 50–200 mg/day
   **Cyclosporine-A = 3.5–5 mg/kg/day
   **Hydroxychloroquine = 200–400 mg/day
   **Rituximab (RA protocol) can be used in relapsing subtype.

- The prognosis of cLCV is usually good. However, one report showed 50 percent of cases achieved complete remission at six to twelve months.

> ##A chronic course of cLCV is related to: positive history of arthralgia, positive cryoglobulins, and no history of fever.

★Vasculitis associated with systemic diseases:-

>>There is a group of vasculitic diseases that occurs secondarily to underlying systemic rheumatic diseases like:

^^*Lupus vasculitis,* and
^^*Rheumatoid vasculitis.*

===>In this part, we will discuss each disease separately in a brief way to have an idea about such complications arising from systemic disorders.

Lupus Vasculitis:

*Introduction:

- SLE is a chronic multisystem autoimmune disease causing different clinical manifestations via immune complex deposition in various organs including blood vessels with different sizes.
- Lupus vasculitis occurs in about 11–36 percent of the patients diagnosed with SLE.
- The pathogenesis of lupus vasculitis depends on: (A) deposition of immune complex in segments of blood vessels, (B) production of pathogenic antibodies like anti-endothelial cells antibodies that can bind to different antigens and causing vascular destruction, (C) presence of ANCA antibodies in some of lupus patients, and (D) as a result of release of high influx of these antibodies, monocytes activation will happen with production of different inflammatory cytokines causing vascular injury.
- Cutaneous vasculitis is the dominant subtype of lupus vasculitis, followed by visceral involvement.

*Clinical manifestations of *lupus vasculitis*:

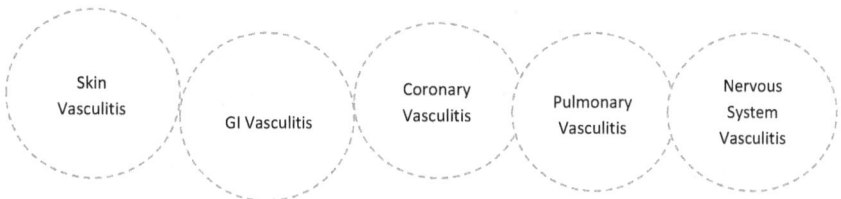

#Cutaneous Vasculitis: *The patients can present with-*

- Papulonodular lesions,
- Palpable purpura,
- Digital infarction,
- Non-blanchable multiple dots lesions appear over palmar surface (most of patients),
- Panniculitis,

- Splinter hemorrhage, and
- Livedo reticularis if these lesions are associated with tender nodular lesions.

#*Gastrointestinal Vasculitis: The patients can present with-*

- Picture of mesenteric vasculitis (MV) affecting superior mesenteric artery, mainly Ileum and jejunum are frequently involved.
- The patients can have: diffuse abdominal pain, vomiting, bloody stool with distended abdomen.
- MV occurs among lupus patients who have active disease in form of lymphopenia, thrombocytopenia, or NPSLE.
- CT abdomen and pelvis can detect mesenteric inflammation by: positive diffuse bowel wall thickening (target sign) and engorgement of mesenteric blood vessels (comb sign).
- Surgical team should be involved early (in less than twenty-four hours) to help in management beside initiation of strong immunosuppressive therapies.

#*Coronary Vasculitis: The patients can present with-*

- There is a higher prevalence of myocardial infarction (MI) among patients with SLE.
- The pathology can be due to atherosclerosis or thrombosis, and may result from vasculitis.
- It happens in most of the cases in the absence of systemic active disease.
- Coronary angiography is useful for diagnosis: isolated segmental involvement with tapering +\- coronary ectasia. (Opinion from a cardiologist is precious!)

#*Pulmonary Vasculitis: The patients can present with-*

- Pulmonary hemorrhage among lupus patients may be either due to systemic inflammation without vasculitis (BLAND) or due to capillaritis.
- Hemoptysis and shortness of breath are frequent symptoms among these patients.

CLINICAL NOTES IN VASCULITIC DISEASES

- It is usually occurring in systemic active disease: lupus nephritis concomitantly.
- High resolution CT chest, bronchoscopy, and BAL are helpful for diagnosis.

#Nervous System Vasculitis: *The patients can present with-*

- Cerebral vessels vasculitis is infrequently seen among patients with lupus.
- A picture of stroke, cerebral cognitive syndrome, myelopathy can arise from thrombosis, neuronal inflammation, or due to vasculitis.
- It is challenging to detect vasculitis in CNS vasculature. However, MRI/MRA CNS can show picture of vasculitis.

>>*Lupus vasculitis occurs in systemic active disease with manifestations like:*

- *Constitutional symptoms like fever, weight loss, and fatigue.*
- *Positive history for livedo reticularis   -Positive anti-SSB/La antibody.*

*Management:

- Cutaneous vasculitic lesions can be treated with: low-dose steroid and dapsone or thalidomide. Anti-malarial therapy should be used in proper dose.
- Mesenteric vasculitis can be treated with: pulse steroid IV followed by high dose of steroid and cyclophosphamide, followed by MMF or azathioprine.
- Cardiac involvement can be treated with: high dose steroid, +\- pulse therapy, and immunosuppressive therapies like MMF, CYC, etc.
- Pulmonary vasculitis can be treated with: pulse steroid IV followed by high dose of steroid, IV cyclophosphamide, PLEX, and IVIG.

>>>*Rituximab can be used in some cases, and also IVIG may show benefits.*

Rheumatoid Vasculitis (RV):

*Introduction:

- RV is considered a part of extra-articular manifestations that occur among patients diagnosed with rheumatoid arthritis (RA).
- Its prevalence started to decrease upon initiation of newer agents used for management of RA. Its prevalence is estimated to be ~ 1–5 percent.
- RV can involve different sizes of blood vessels, mainly small followed by medium-sized vascular beds.
- Risk factors for RV development based on a case-control study that included eighty-six patients:

(A)Male gender,
(B)Early onset of (RA) diagnosis,
(C)Longer disease duration ~ ten years,
(D)Current smoker at RA diagnosis,
(E)Joints damage (positive erosion),
(F)History of joints replacement,
(G)Presence of rheumatoid nodules, and
(H)Positive history of cerebrovascular disease or peripheral artery disease.

- The prognosis of RV is poor, with 26–50 percent mortality rate at five years, and the survival rate declines either by damaged blood vessels causing organs damage or by strong effects of immunosuppressants.

*Pathogenesis:

- The pathogenesis of RV depends on many factors present among patients diagnosed with this phenomenon including seropositive (RA) patients with genetic susceptibility by positive HLA –DRB1, and rheumatoid antibodies may play a role in RV occurrence.
- The relevance between RV and positive rheumatoid antibodies like RF and anti-CCP released from the ability to form immune-complex deposits that can manifest with vascular inflammation. However, positivity of rheumatoid antibodies among patients with RA doesn't have a magnitude for

appearance of RV. This is actually explaining why not all RA patients with positive rheumatoid antibodies will develop RV.
- During presence of active inflammatory cascade in RA, the production of cytokines will be stimulated with possibility of immune-complex deposition, monocytes and neutrophils will be activated. *Vascular inflammation will happen!*

★Clinical assessment:

- Cutaneous vasculitis: the most common form of RV, and the patients can present with-

(A) palpable purpura,
(B) ulcers,
(c) digital necrosis or infarction,
(D) livedo reticularis.

- Peripheral nervous system involvement: the second most affected organ by RV, and the patients can present with-

(A) distal sensory polyneuropathy,
(B) distal sensorimotor polyneuropathy,
(C) mononeuritis multiplex.

>>Other visceral organs can be infrequently by RV, like CNS, heart, Bowel, and kidneys.

★Investigations:

- Anemia of chronic disease is seen in ~ 55 percent, while leukocytosis is noticed in ~27 percent, and high count of platelets observed in ~ 17 percent.
- High ESR or High CRP seen at ~ 67 percent.
- Deep punch skin biopsy: to decide if it is related to small or medium vessels pathology.
- Electromyography or nerve conduction velocity (EMG\NCV): to recognize what is the nature of this nerve injury.
- Muscle and nerve biopsy: to see any vascular inflammatory infiltrate.

*Management:

- The treatment of RV depends on the organs influenced by vasculitis.
- In most of cases of RV, the treatment is composed of: steroid (0.5–1 mg/kg), tapered after two to four weeks, and immunosuppressant therapies.
- Mild organs manifestations like skin or mild nerve: steroid and MTX or azathioprine.
- The use of cyclophosphamide (CYC) or rituximab (RTX) is advised when there are major affected organs.
- Use of biological drugs like: TNF inhibitors which may be a valid option for controlling RV. However, we have to be cautious that TNFi can promote vasculitis.
- Also, abatacept can be used for managing patients diagnosed with RV.

*Monitoring:

- Development of RV among patients with RA is considered a poor prognostic phenomenon.
- Follow-up after six months: *38 percent* will achieve complete remission, *52 percent* will have partial improvement, and *10 percent* will not get any improvement.
- The relapse rate is high, reaching up to 36 percent. So we have to follow the patients closely to be sure that these individuals are not having any recurred symptoms

*Vasculitis Mimickers:

>>>*These are vascular disorders not occurring due to primary autoimmune phenomenon and may participate with genuine vasculitis diseases in some clinical and radiological features.*

>>>*It is important to identify these disorders early to avoid nonmandatory administration of immunosuppressants.*

CLINICAL NOTES IN VASCULITIC DISEASES

>>>*In this chapter, we will discuss some examples of vasculitis mimickers based on the size of involved blood vessels.*

^Clinical cases can be a mimicker for (LVV)	^Clinical cases can be a mimicker for (MVV)	^Clinical cases can be a mimicker for (SVV)
1-Infectious aortitis	1-Fibromuscular dysplasia	1-Infectious causes like: HIV, Aspergillosis, severe bacterial pneumonia and sepsis, COVID-19-related systemic inflammation
2-Atherosclerosis	2-Segmental arterial mediolysis	
3-IgG4-related diseases	3-Calciphylaxis	2-Drug eruption or DRESS
4-Genetic disorders like: Marfan syndrome or EDS	4-Mycotic aneurysms	3-ITP, TTP, APS
		4-Warfarin-induced skin necrosis
5-Relapsing polychondritis		5-Paraproteinemia or amyloidosis
6-Erdheim-Chester disease		6-Hypereosinophilic syndrome (HES)

Conditions may be a mimicker for (LVV):

> *Infectious aortitis:*

A- Tuberculous aortitis || True aneurysm (Rasmussen's lesion) and pseudoaneurysm

B- Syphilitic aortitis || Ascending thoracic aortic aneurysm or aortic insufficiency

> *IgG4 – related disease: Autoimmune fibro-inflammatory disease*

Abdominal aortic aneurysm with aortitis +\- retroperitoneal fibrosis. It is characterized by lymphoplasmacytic infiltration, storiform fibrosis, and obliterative phlebitis.

> *Genetic disorders:*

A- Marfan syndrome: Autosomal dominant disorder caused by mutation in *fibrillin-1* gene. The patients will have be tall with long arm span, high-arched palate, ectopia lentis, spontaneous pneumothorax, and aortic root dilation.

B- Ehlers-Danlos syndrome (EDS): Autosomal dominant heritable connective tissue disorder characterized by mutation in gene responsible for type I or III collagen. Patients diagnosed with EDS can have joints hypermobility, skin hyper elasticity, and hollow organs rupture.

> *Erdheim-Chester's disease:*

Non-Langerhans histiocytic disease with multisystem symptoms: The patients will have osteosclerotic bony lesions with retroperitoneal infiltration, periorbital disease, and cardiac pseudotumors.

#Conditions may be a mimicker for MVV:

>*Fibromuscular dysplasia (FMD):*

It is an idiopathic noninflammatory vasculopathy that occurs mainly among women with age ranging from their twenties thirties. The disease involves renal arteries mostly, and other vascular territories can be affected like carotid and intracerebral arteries. Clinical manifestations of FMD are broad, like hypertension, headache, tinnitus, dizziness, AKI, CVA, and MI. The radiological appearance of FMD is looking with focal or multifocal (strings on beads), alternating with stenosis and aneurysms.

> *Segmental arterial mediolysis (SAM):*

It is non-atherosclerotic, noninflammatory disease with unknown etiology associated with degeneration of the medial layers of arteries. It occurs in both genders equally with age from fifties to sixties. Mesenteric arteries are commonly affected. However, renal and retroperitoneal vasculatures might be involved. The radiological features of SAM: classical strings on beads with alternating stenosis and dilation with occlusive lesions—thrombi. The feature that differentiates between FMD and SAM radiologically is occlusive lesions among patients with SAM. Dangerous manifestations like dissection and hemorrhage may happen as sequelae of SAM.

> *Calciphylaxis:*

Calciphylaxis or calcific uremic arteriolopathy (CUA): It is a phenomenon usually occurring among patients with advanced chronic kidney disease due to abnormal calcium-phosphate homeostasis. The lesions commonly affect lower limbs with necrotic, black painful tissue. The pathological specimen from CUA showed: calcified deposits in the medial layers of dermal and subcutaneous arterioles. This cutaneous lesions are associated with higher morbidity and mortality.

> *Mycotic aneurysms:*

It is an aneurysm formed as a complication from severe infective endocarditis due to bacterial migration into vasa vasorum, causing wall thinning with aneurismal formation at the point of bifurcation of vascular tree.

#Conditions may be a mimicker for (SVV):

> *Severe infections like severe pneumonia with sepsis*

In case of severe infections causing septicemia, multi-organ failure will occur as a result of high amount of inflammatory cytokines. Pulmonary failure and renal injury may be sequelae for septicemia with a picture closely mimicking for vasculitides causing pulmonary-renal syndrome.

>Drugs eruption:

Maculopapular rash that spread diffusely after usage of specific medications like antibiotics. This rash tend to fade after stopping offending medication. However, systemic phenomenon with eosinophilia and systemic manifestations can happen.

>ITP, TTP, APS:

A- ITP: It is an autoimmune disorder in which there is platelets destruction, and the patients can develop purpuric-like rash.

B- TTP: Subtype of MAHA associated with thrombocytopenia and thrombotic manifestations. It is usually occurring due to abnormal function of ADAMTS 13 that leads to abnormal cleavage of vWF.

C- APS: Anti-phospholipid antibodies can lead to overt thrombotic events in any vascular bed. But in severe case like CAPS, even microthrombotic disease might occur.

>Warfarin-Induced Skin Necrosis:

It is a type of skin rash rarely occurring among middle-aged obese women being started recently in the first *three to six days* on warfarin for treating PE or DVT. This rash happened due to abnormal fast reduction in the level of protein C *natural anticoagulant* that lead to microthrombotic cutaneous lesion that should be treated with IV heparin and surgical debridement, +\- FFP administration.

COVID-19 related vascular inflammation (A novel mimicker):

- COVID-19 infection: It is a subtype of respiratory viral infection (SARS-CoV-2) that appeared for the first time in China in December 2019. Then the virus started to spread worldwide to become a *pandemic crisis*.

CLINICAL NOTES IN VASCULITIC DISEASES

- There was a thought that COVID-19 infection is usually affecting respiratory tract. However, many systemic inflammatory manifestations started to develop.
- Vascular disease among patients with COVID-19 infection is occurring mainly due to several mechanisms, like pulmonary intravascular coagulopathy, PE, DVT, and arterial thrombosis. Additionally, hypoxemia, viral dissemination, and immobility can attribute for vascular injury among infected patients.
- There are many patterns of vascular damage related to COVID-19 infection:

A- *Cutaneous vasculitis-related to COVID-19 infection:* The lesions appear mainly in the dorsal surface of the toes with rounded erythematous chilblain-like disease. The pathology stands behind skin vasculitis differs, dependent on disease severity. These manifestation can appear in the patients with mild respiratory disease with minimal vasculitic changes. In opposite to the patients who have severe lung disease, cutaneous lesions mainly arise from severe thromboembolic disease causing multi-organ dysfunction.

B- *Myocardial involvement or Kawasaki-like disease related to COVID-19 infection:* The young patients with mild or no symptoms of COVID-19 infection may present with Kawasaki-like picture without formation of coronary artery aneurysm. This could be related to endotheliitis caused by COVID-19 viral particles. Many patients infected with severe COVID-19 disease can develop severe myopericarditis and can present with high cardiac enzymes.

C- *Arterial and venous thrombosis among patients with severe COVID-19 disease:* Severe disease may be associated with large DVT or arterial thrombosis in form of digital gangrene. Thrombosis in the pulmonary venular tree is originating from severe inflammation resulting in a higher level of inflammatory cytokines with enhanced activity of inflammatory cells *(neutrophils)* that leads to release of procoagulant factor—*immunothromboembolism.* Systemic thrombotic phase tends to correlate with viremia that can induce vascular damage. As a sequela for this process, transmigration of emboli might happen from the heart into various arterial beds.

D- *CNS vascular damage-related to COVID-19 infection:* Among patients with severe COVID-19 infection, ischemic cerebral events (e.g. stroke) may appear either due to microthrombi or related to cerebral vascular inflammation. Other neurological syndromes like encephalopathy and muscle injury can appear.

E- *Other organs can have angiitis in patients with COVID-19 infection:* Infarction in the liver, spleen, and kidneys might occur due to systemic occlusive microthrombi.

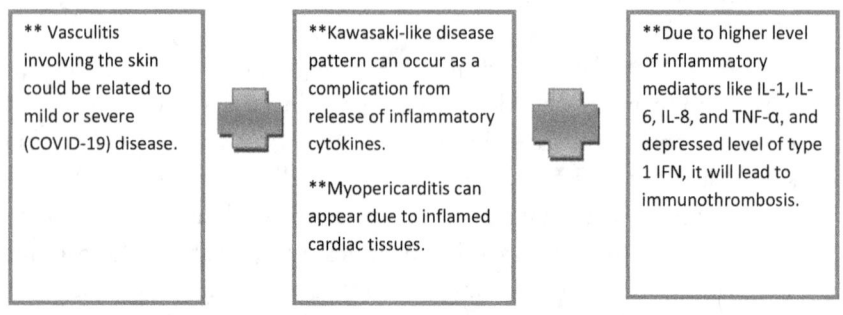

Patterns of vascular injury-related to COVID-19 infection

(3) THE THIRD CHAPTER

THERAPEUTIC AGENTS IN MANAGEMENT OF VASCULITIS

Common medications used in treatment of vasculitic patients:

> *Glucocorticoids*
> *Conventional synthetic DMARDs (csDMARDs)*
> (Methotrexate)
> *Regular immunosuppressive medications*
> (Azathioprine or mycophenolate mofetil *MMF*)
> *Biological therapies*
> (Anti-TNF-α, tocilizumab, rituximab, mepolizumab)
> *Cytotoxic agent*
> (Cyclophosphamide)
> *Other miscellaneous drugs*
> (Colchicine, dapsone, cyclosporine-A, apremilast)
> *A brief talk about PLASMA EXCHANGE,* PLEX *and* IVIG

>Glucocorticoids (GCs):

- GCs are potent anti-inflammatory agents used in the treatment of different rheumatic diseases, including vasculitis >>> for induction of remission, then tapering gradually.
- Mechanism of action:

^ *GCs molecules have the ability to pass easily through different cell membranes.*
^ *GCs exert their actions via binding to their receptors intra-cellularly GCRs.*

- When GCs-GCRs interaction occurs, this complex will diffuse inside the nucleus of different cells, and this combined molecule will bind to glucocorticoids response elements (GREs).
- Each GREs has an association with different genes responsible for stimulation or suppression of transcription (nucleic acid or protein synthesis).
- So, as consequences of this process: suppression the synthesis of (phospholipase A2 enzyme) that plays a role in production of different inflammatory mediators
- Additionally, GCs can inhibit the synthesis of cyclo-oxygenase-2 enzyme by inhibition of the gene, and GCs can decrease the release of TNF-α and different leukotriens.
- GCs can enhance the activity of Annexin A1. As a result of that, the release of prostaglandins will be decreased and migration of neutrophils toward the site of inflammation will be impaired.

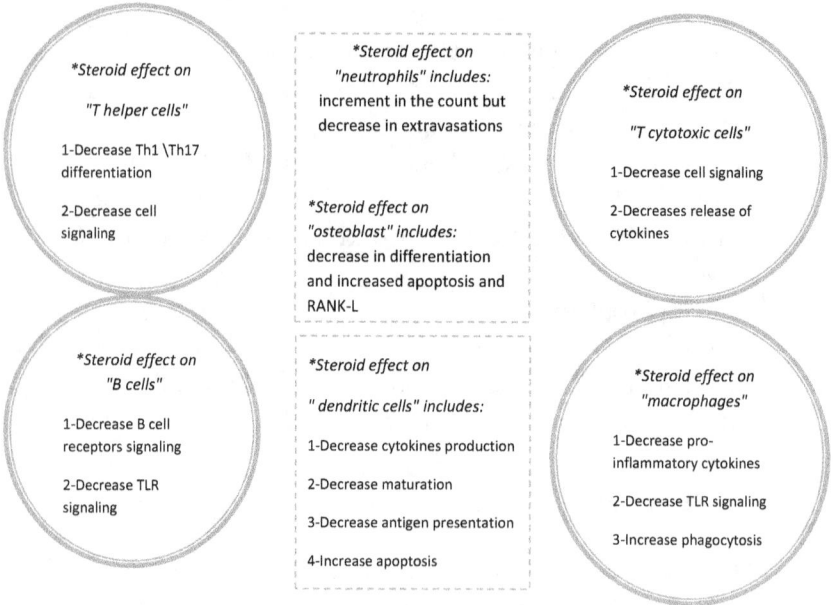

- Dose of glucocorticoid (GCs) therapy:

* *Low dose*: ≤ 7.5 mg PO daily
* *Medium dose*: > 7.5 mg PO daily to ≤ 30 mg PO daily
* *High dose*: > 30 mg PO daily to ≤ 100 mg PO daily (To induce remission in most of vasculitic cases and during active phase.)

* *Pulse therapy*: 15 mg/kg/day (IV route) for three to five days (used in severe cases like pulmonary hemorrhage or RPGN) >>> Check potassium level before infusion as it can exacerbate arrhythmia (Steroid can cause low potassium level!).

**Side effects of long-standing glucocorticoids therapy (GCs):

- Cushingoid appearance: moon face, striae, buffalo hump, and obesity
- Hypothalamic-pituitary-adrenal axis suppression
- Hypertension
- Glucose intolerance
- Peptic ulcer disease
- Acne
- Hirsutism
- Insomnia
- Atrophy of the skin or bruises
- Psychiatric symptoms
- Decreased bone density
- Muscle atrophy
- Cataract or glaucoma
- Increased risk of infections >>> Immunosuppression *(PCP, viral, or bacterial)*

> **Conventional synthetic disease modifying antirheumatic drugs (csDMARDs):**

***Methotrexate (MTX)*: It is a drug applying its effect by two important mechanisms-

*Inhibition of dihydrofolate reductase will lead to decrease the amount of tetrahydrobiopterin which can result in enhanced the response of apoptosis in T-cells >>> attenuating inflammatory activity.

*Inhibition of aminoimidazole-4-carboxamide ribonucleotide (AICAR) transformylase enzyme. So this action will cause rise in AICAR level intracellularly, and adenosine level will increase, resulting in suppression of immune response.

- MTX will cause an increment in the level of adenosine, and this rise in adenosine will have many effects on inflammatory cells: (1) inhibits neutrophilic adhesion and NET formation; (2) inhibits T-cells activation; (3) increases barrier integrity in endothelial cells; (4) prevents osteoclast differentiation; and (5) enhances the level of T- regulatory cells (Treg).
- Dosing of MTX drug: 10–25 mg weekly (PO or SC) and folic acid (used as steroid sparing agent in different subtypes of vasculitis).
- Side effects of MTX therapy: (A) bone marrow suppression, (B) liver injury, and (C) lung injury (pneumonitis), (D) mucositis, (E) GI upset with nausea and vomiting, and (F) hair loss.

>>>Methotrexate is contraindicated during pregnancy (*teratogenic* and should be stopped for twelve weeks before conception)!

>>>Be careful! Use adjusted dose among patients who have renal impairment.

>>>Follow CBC with differentials and LFTs closely in the beginning, then monthly and every three to six months thereafter.

==

> **Regular immunosuppressive medications:**

**Azathioprine*: It is a prodrug that inhibits purine synthesis by production of thioguanine nucleotide. This drug is used as steroid sparing agent in different vasculitic disorders.

- Dose of azathioprine: 2 mg/kg daily divided into two doses. Among patients with Behcet's disease (BD), the proper dose is ~ 2.5 mg/kg/day. Increase the dose gradually after four to six weeks to have a chance to check CBC with Differentials or LFTs.
- Side effects of azathioprine: (1) bone marrow suppression, (2) liver injury, (3) pancreatitis, (4) photosensitivity, (5) increase the risk for infection, (6) it can decrease the anticoagulation

effect of warfarin, and (7) hypersensitivity reaction: fever, myalgia, rise in LFT, and skin rash.
- Measurement of TPMT enzyme can be requested, however is not routinely recommended.
- Due to its influence on lymphocyte, azathioprine increases the risk of viral infections like VZV and CMV.
- It's a safe drug to be used during pregnancy and breastfeeding!

==

**Mycophenolate Mofetil (MMF): It is a prodrug that inhibits inosine-5-monophosphate dehydrogenase enzyme (I5MPD). The result will be prevention of de novo synthesis of guanosine nucleotide [Its effect on both T & B cells] >>> Used as steroid sparing agent in some of vasculitic cases.

- The suitable dose of (MMF) is ranging between 2–3 g PO daily in two divided doses. The dose will be increased gradually every seven days to reach the proper dose, and to check the labs (CBC with differentials or LFTs) more frequently in the beginning, then periodically. *(Don't combine MMF with antacid. MMF absorption will be lower.*
- Side effects of MMF: (1) bone marrow suppression, (2) GI intolerance, (3) liver injury, and (4) increase the risk of infections like CMV, PCP, and JC-associated PML. *(MMF is teratogenic and contraindicated during pregnancy should be stopped six weeks before conception!)*

==

> **Biological therapies-**

**Anti-TNF α: They are biological agents (monoclonal antibodies) targeting (TNF-α) cytokines that rise in different inflammatory disorders including vasculitis.

- There are five drugs under this group: infliximab (IV route), adalimumab (SC route), etanercept (SC route), certolizumab (SC route), and golimumab (SC route).

- The proper dose of Infliximab = 5 mg/kg IV at zero, two, and six weeks, then every eight weeks, and the dose of adalimumab = 40 mg SC q for two weeks, while the dose of etanercept = 50 mg SC weekly (Don't use etanercept for cases with uveitis or IBD).
- Side effects of anti-TNF α: (1) Increase the risk of bacterial infections, especially respiratory tract infections, (2) it can cause TB reactivation in the first three to six months, (3) it can lead to Hepatitis B reactivation & (4) Injection site reaction & (5) anti – TNF α can disturb CBC, (6) these drugs can induce autoimmune phenomenon like lupus, PsO, etc., and (7) don't use it among patients with congestive heart failure or demyelinating disorders.
- Anti-TNF α are used in: Takayasu arteritis, Behcet's disease, polyarteritis nodosa, and some refractory cases of Kawasaki disease.
- Anti-TNF α are safe medications during pregnancy and breastfeeding!
- Screen the patients for TB and hepatitis serology before initiation of these drugs!
- Infliximab can cause infusion reaction: fever, headache, rash, and anaphylaxis. It is reasonable to premedicate the patients with acetaminophen, steroid, and antihistamine drugs.

===

**Tocilizumab: It is a humanized monoclonal antibody that can bind to IL-6 receptor.

- The dose of tocilizumab = 8 mg/kg IV monthly, while the dose can be taken via SC route = 162 mg SC weekly.
- Side effects of Tocilizumab: (1) bone marrow suppression (neutropenia or thrombocytopenia), (2) injection site reaction, (3) dyslipidemia, (4) liver injury, (5) increase the risk of infections (URTI), and (6) don't use it among patients who have history of diverticulitis. It can lead to GI perforation.
- Follow CBC with differentials or LFTs monthly, then every two to three months, while the lipid panel can be ordered after two months from initiation of therapy, then every three to six months.

- Tocilizumab used among patients with LVV, such as giant cell arteritis (GCA), and in some cases diagnosed with Behcet's disease (BD).
- It cannot be used during pregnancy and breastfeeding *(no data)!* So avoid it!

===

**Rituximab (RTX): It is a chimeric monoclonal antibody that binds against *CD20* present on developing B cells before going to the stage of plasma cells. It is used for induction and maintenance of remission in some types of vasculitis (AAV).

- Dose of (RTX): *RA protocol* 1g IV two doses separated by two weeks, then every six months. There is an additional protocol that is called *lymphoma protocol* in which the dose of RTX will be 375 mg/m2 IV weekly for four weeks, then every six months.
- Side effects of (RTX): (1) Hypogammaglobulinemia, (2) late-onset neutropenia, (3) reactivation of hepatitis B, (4) Increase the risk for JC-associated PML, (5) liver injury, and (6) infusion reaction with chills, rash, anaphylaxis, HTN, and myocardial infarction. So you have to stop the infusion. It is valuable to premedicate the patients with IV methylprednisolone, acetaminophen, and antihistamine drugs.
- It cannot be used during pregnancy! So avoid the use of RTX during conception.
- Check CBC with differentials or LFTs and immunoglobulins level before starting RTX, then periodically.

===

**Mepolizumab: It is a humanized monoclonal antibody works against IL-5. So it will impair maturation, recruitment, and survival of eosinophils.

- Dose of mepolizumab: 300 mg SC monthly in case with EGPA.
- Side effects of Mepolizumab: (1) Headache, (2) Injection site reaction, (3) Back pain and fatigue, (4) Increase risk of VZV infection, and (5) pruritus.

– *No* data about its use in pregnancy. (Avoid it.)

===

> **Cytotoxic agents:**

⋆⋆*Cyclophosphamide (CYC)*: It is a cytotoxic medication *prodrug* that should be converted into active form: phosphoramide mustard, and this active substance will cause *DNA* alkylation, with cross linking of *DNA* and decrease *DNA* generation.

- The dose of CYC: Oral route = 2mg/kg/day, and IV route in which can be given either monthly for six doses = 500–750 mg /m2 monthly for six months, or as in CYCLOPS regimen = 15mg/kg every two weeks for three doses, then every three weeks for three to six months.
- Side effects of CYC:

(1) Bone marrow suppression: leukopenia or neutropenia >>> to check CBC with differential before infusion, then after seven to ten days from the dose.
(2) Decrease the fertility rate: leuprolide should be given for women ten days prior to the IV dose.
(3) Increase the risk of infection PCP: TMP-SMX to be prescribed as prophylaxis during treatment.
(4) Hemorrhagic cystitis: due to accumulation of toxic metabolite (ACROLINE) in the urinary bladder. So aggressive IV hydration pre- and post-infusion is recommended and MESNA therapy.
(5) Increase the risk of malignancy: especially among older patients, smokers, and received high cumulative dose of CYC. IV route is associated with lower cumulative dose.
(6) Pneumonitis can occur in some patients using CYC.
(7) PRES syndrome after IV infusion (CYC).
(8) Hair loss.
(9) GI intolerance.
(10) It is contraindicated during pregnancy and breastfeeding.

- Check CBC with differentials or LFTs, renal profile, hepatitis serology, and quantiFERON-TB before starting CYC.
- CYC is used for induction of remission in different subtypes of vasculitis.

==

> **Other miscellaneous drugs:**

**Colchicine: It is a drug that inhibits microtubule assembly, preventing neutrophilic migration toward the site of inflammation.

- The dose of Colchicine: 0.5 mg PO twice a day.
- It is used in treatment crystals-induced arthropathy, and regularly used among patients diagnosed with BD.
- Side effects of colchicines: (1) GI intolerance like nausea, vomiting, and diarrhea; (2) bone marrow suppression; (3) neuromyopathy; (4) rash; (5) hemorrhagic gastritis; (6) circulatory failure and shock; (7) respiratory insufficiency; and (8) liver injury.
- Check CBC with differentials, LFTs, or kidneys function. Use adjusted dose in relation to CrCl.
- Be careful! Colchicine has many drug-drug interaction. So be aware before prescribing any medication in patients using colchicine (e.g., clarithromycin, etc.).

==

**Dapsone: It is a drug that works as free radicals scavenger. Anti-inflammatory property (used in some cases with BD and some conditions with cutaneous vasculitis).

- The dose of dapsone: 50–200 mg PO daily, and the dose increased gradually each ten days.
- Check G6PD level before initiating this therapy!
- Side effects of dapsone: (1) leukopenia, (2) liver injury, (3) hemolysis, (4) methemoglobinemia, and (5) neuropathy.

==

**Cyclosporine-A (CsA)*: It is a medication that belongs to the family of calcineurin inhibitor that inhibits cell division of lymphocytes (used in some symptoms of Behcet's disease).

- The dose of CsA: 2.5–4 mg/kg daily, divided into two doses per day, and the dose should be titrated up gradually. *(It's safe to be used in pregnancy.)*
- Side effects of CsA: (1) hypertension, (2) hirsutism, (3) hyperkalemia, (4) neurotoxicity, (5) renal impairment, and (6) dyslipidemia.

**Apremilast*: This drug acts by inhibition of phosphodiesterase-4 enzyme (PDE4). This leads to increase in intracellular level of cAMP which has anti-inflammatory effect by reducing synthesis of TNF-α, IL-12, and IL-23.

- The dose of apremilast: 10 mg PO OD for one day, then increase the dose by 10 mg daily till reaching active dose of ~ 30 mg PO twice daily.
- Side effects of apremilast: (1) diarrhea, (2) Headache, (3) weight loss, and (4) depression?
- It is used among patients with BD who have refractory mucocutaneous manifestations, and it can be used during active infection *(not immunosuppressive medication)*!
- Adjust the dose of apremilast if CrCl < 30ml/min/m2!

==

>> A brief talk about intravenous immunoglobulins administration (IVIG):

- *Intravenous immunoglobulins (IVIG)*: The use of immunoglobulins in management of vasculitis is not commonly seen. However, patients with Kawasaki disease (KD) should receive IVIG once diagnosis is established.
- The dose of (IVIG) = either 2g/kg to be given over ten to twelve hours or ~ 400 mg/kg/day for five days.
- IVIG can work as an immunosuppressive modality especially in case of vasculitis with an active infection in which other

CLINICAL NOTES IN VASCULITIC DISEASES

  immunosuppressive drugs are contraindicated (AAV with pulmonary hemorrhage and active infection).
- Side effects of IVIG: (1) infusion reaction: fever, chills, chest tightness, anaphylaxis, hypotension; (2) back pain; (3) headache; (4) aseptic meningitis; (5) thrombosis; and (6) some components in IVIG can cause AKI.
- It is advised to premedicate the patients with steroid, acetaminophen, and antihistamine drugs to reduce the risk of infusion reaction.
- Always start the infusion with low dose and slow infusion, then increase the infusion rate gradually.

===

> **A brief talk about *Therapeutic Plasma Exchange* (PLEX or TPE):**

- PLEX: It is an exchange modality used in management of different cases of vasculitis.
- The aim of doing PLEX: (A) to remove pathological antibodies responsible for disease occurrence, and (B) to wash out pathological inflammatory substances like adhesion molecules and complements.
- The prescription of plasma exchange: to exchange one plasma volume (30–60 ml/kg actual body weight) in each session with replacement of fluid with albumin 5 percent +\- saline. Total number of sessions = seven sessions over fourteen days.

**IV methylprednisolone versus PLEX in vasculitis MEPEX trial: It is a trial done earlier in 2007 to describe any role for plasma exchange in managing the patients with AAV. This study included 137 patients with severe renal disease with creatinine > 500 μmol/L or requiring dialysis at presentation with a high BVAS ~21 and a high CRP~93 mg/dl. The patients were randomized to receive either IV methylprednsiolone or seven sessions of PLEX. All of these arms received oral cyclophosphamide and oral prednisolone. The results from this study showed that patients who received PLEX attained more recovery of renal function at three months and less requirement of dialysis at twelve months without any impact on mortality.

Plasma exchange and glucocorticoids dosing in treatment of AAV PEXIVAS trial: It is a recent trial published in NEJM in 2020, and this study was designed by 2*2 factor design to describe the arms either with or without PLEX and either with standard dose or reduced dose of glucocorticoids. About 704 patients were included with Crcl < 50 ml/min/m2 (Cr~ 330μmol/L), and patients with pulmonary hemorrhage also included. All patients received either cyclophosphamide or rituximab, plus prednisolone in standard versus reduced strategies. The results released from this study showed PLEX doesn't add any positive effect on ESRD or deaths. However, reduced dose strategy was associated with lower risk of infections compared to standard regimen.

>>>There are many points that can explain the difference in the outcomes between these studies. This is actually not closing the door about usage of PLEX in management (AAV), in opposite the trials to identify who are the patients may get benefit from PLEX??

##PLEX may be an option in specific circumstances of *AAV*:

1– Patients with dual positivity ANCA and anti-GBM.
2– Patients with picture of *RPGN* with a high level of creatinine and no chronic changes in renal biopsy.
3– Patients who required renal replacement therapy acutely and the biopsy revealed high number of glomeruli with crescent formation.
4– Patients didn't respond to initial immunosuppressive therapies.

^^*Some important complications from PLEX:*

1– Related to vascular line: bleeding, infection, or thrombosis
2– Anaphylactic reaction
3– Disturbance of coagulation profile
4– Metabolic derangement: metabolic alkalosis or hypocalcaemia
5– Hypotension: due to circulatory hypoperfusion

**Examples of vasculitic cases may need PLEX to control disease activity:

A-HBV-associated PAN
B-Severe cases of cryoglobulinemic vasculitis
C-Specific conditions of AAV >>> controversial!

(4) THE FOURTH CHAPTER

TEST YOURSELF (SHORT REAL CASES)

Case 1: This is a seventy-one-year-old female, known case of diabetes mellitus on oral hypoglycemic agents, presented to ED with history of temporal headache started one week ago. (Approach for GCA vasculitis.)

Case 2: This is a thirty-one-year-old male, known case of old pulmonary TB treated four years ago, presented to ED with history of neck pain developed six weeks ago associated with history of subjective fever and generalized fatigability. CT-angiogram of the neck showed left subclavian artery narrowing. (Approach for TA vasculitis.)

Case 3: This is a forty-three-year-old male, presented to ED with history of numbness in legs with digital ulcers developed two months ago. The patient has constitutional symptoms in form of fever and weight loss. (Approach for PAN vasculitis.)

Case 4: This is a forty-year-old lady, not known to have any medical illness. She had been referred from outside hospital with history of epistaxis, chronic cough, and impaired renal function with serum creatinine = 150μ mol/L. (Approach for GPA vasculitis.)

Case 5: Fifty-year-old woman, known case of diabetes mellitus and bronchial asthma diagnosed twenty years ago. The patient admitted under the team of general internal medicine with history of shortness of breath and productive cough with tinged blood. (Approach for EGPA vasculitis.)

Case 6: This is a twenty-eight-year-old male, referred from ophthalmology clinic as the patient developed sudden blurred vision in the right eye. Upon examination, the patient has panuveal inflammation. (Approach for Behcet's disease.)

Case 7: Forty-eight-year-old gentleman, medically free, admitted under care of neurology team for work-up regarding multiple attacks of strokes, cognitive impairment, and headache for four months. (Approach for PACNS vasculitis.)

Case 8: Sixteen-year-old girl, presented to ED with history of bilateral lower limbs purpuric rash and fever developed over one week. (Approach for cLCV vasculitis.)

CASE 9: Thirty-six-year-old woman, medically free, presented to ED with history of purpuric rash over the legs that became diffuse over the forearms through two weeks, with history of arthritis involving knee joints. (Approach for HSP vasculitis.)

Case 10: Forty-two-year-old woman, known case of SLE maintained currently on hydroxychloroquine 200 milligrams daily. She came to ED with history of severe diffuse abdominal pain, vomiting, and diarrhea for the last three days. (Approach for lupus-related vasculitis.)

REFERENCES

Barile-Fabris, L., M. F. Hernandez-Cabrera, and J. A. Barragan-Garfias. 2014. "Vasculitis in Systemic Lupus Erythematosus." *Curr Rheumatol Rep.*

Bartels and Bridges. 2011. "Rheumatoid Vasculitis: Vanishing Menace or Target for New Treatments?" *Curr Rheumatol Rep.*

Beuker, Carolin, et al. 2018. "Primary Angiitis of the central nervous system: diagnosis and treatment." *Therapeutic Advances in Neurological Disorders.*

Birnbaum, Julius and David B. Hellmann. 2009. "Primary Angiitis of the Central Nervous System." *Arch Neurol.*

Chung, Sharon A., et al. 2021. "2021 American College of Rheumatology/Vasculitis Foundation Guideline for the Management of Polyarteritis Nodosa." *Arthritis Care & Research.*

Clunie, Dr. Gavin, Dr. Nick Wilkinson, Dr. Elena Nikiiphorou, and Dr. Deepak Jadon. Oxford Handbook Of Rheumatology, Fourth Edition.

Dejaco C. et al. 2018. "EULAR recommendation for the use of imaging in large vessels vasculitis in clinical practice." Ann Rheum Dis.

D'Aguanno V. et al. 2018. "Optimal management of Cogan's syndrome: a multidisciplinary approach." *Journal of Multidisciplinary Healthcare.*

Emmi G. et al. 2019. "Vascular Behcet's syndrome: an update." *Internal and Emergency Medicine.*

Floege, Jurgen and Frank Eitner. 2011. "Current Therapy for IgA Nephropathy." *J Am Soc Nephrol.*

Geetha, Duvuru and Ashley Jefferson. 2019. "ANCA-Associated Vasculitis: Core Curriculum 2020." *Am J Kidney Dis.*

Goglin, Sarah and Sharon A. Chung. 2016. "Current Treatment of Cryoglobulinemic Vasculitis." *Curr Treat Options in Rheum.*

Gornik, Heather L. and Mark A. Creager. 2008. "Aortitis." *Circulation.*

Gota, Carmen E. and Leonard H. Calabrese. 2013. "Diagnosis and treatment of cutaneous leukocytoclastic vasculitis." *Int. J. Clin. Rheumatol.*

Greco A. et al. 2015. "Microscopic polyangiitis: Advances in diagnosis and therapeutic approaches." *Autoimmunity Reviews.*

Groh M. et al. 2015. "Eosinophilic granulomatosis with polyangiitis (Churg-Strauss) (EGPA) Consensus Task Force recommendations for evaluation and management." *European Journal of Internal Medicine.*

Hatemi G. et al. 2018. "2018 update of the EULAR recommendations for the management of Behcet's syndrome." *Ann Rheum Dis.*

Heineke, M.H., et al. 2017. "New insights in the pathogenesis of immunoglobulin A vasculitis (Henoch-Scnlein purpura). *Autoimmunity Reviews.*

Hellmich B. et al. 2019. "2018 Update of the EULAR recommendations for the management of large vessels vasculitis." *Ann Rheum Dis.*

Hellmich B. et al. 2020. "Treatment of Giant Cell Arteritis and Takaysu Arteritis–Current and Future." *Current Rheumatology Reports–Springer.*

Hocevar A. et al. 2019. "Predicting gastrointestinal and renal involvement in adult IgA vasculitis." *Arthritis Research & Therapy.*

International Team for the Revision of the International Criteria for Behcet's Disease (ITR-ICBD). 2014. "International Criteria for Behcet's Disease (ICBD): a collaborative study of 27 countries on the sensitivity and specificity of the new criteria." *Journal of the European Academy of Dermatology and Venereology.*

Jennette et al. 2013. "2012 Revised International Chapel Hill Consensus Conference Nomenclature of Vasculitides." *Arthritis & Rheumatism–ACR.*

Kokturk, Aysin. 2012. "Clinical and Pathological Manifestations with differential Diagnosis in Behcet's Disease." *Pathology Research International-Hindawi.*

Kolkhir P. et al. 2019. "Treatment of urticarial vasculitis: A systematic review." *J Allergy Clin Immunol.*

Low, Candice and Richard Conway. 2019. "Current advances in the treatment of giant cell arteritis: the role of biologics." *Therapeutic Advances in Musculoskeletal Disease.*

Lutalo, Pamela M. K. and David P. D'Cruz. 2014. "Diagnosis and classification of granulomatosis with polyangiitis (aka Wegner's granulomatosis)." *Journal of Autoimmunity.*

Makol, Ashima, et al. 2014. "Vasculitis associated with rheumatoid arthritis: a case-control study." *Oxford Journal.*

Maleszewski, Joseph J. 2015. "Inflammatory ascending aortic disease: Perspective from pathology." *The Journal of Thoracic and Cardiovascular Surgery.*

Marchesi, Alessandra et al. 2021. "Revised recommendations for the Italian Society of Pediatrics about the general management of Kawasaki disease." *Italian Journal of Pediatrics*

Maritati F. et al. 2020. "Adult-onset IgA vasculitis (Henoch-Schonlein): Update on therapy." *Press Med.*

McGonagle, Dennis, et al. 2021. "COVID-19 vasculitis and novel vasculitis mimics." *The Lancet Rheumatol.*

Miller, A., M. Chan, A. Wiik, S. A. Misbah, and R. A. Luqmani. 2010. "An approach to the diagnosis and management of systemic vasculitis." *British Society for Immunology, Clinical & Experimental Immunology.*

Misra, Durga Prasanna Misra, et al. 2019. "Recent advances in the management of Takayasu arteritis." *International Journal of Rheumatic Diseases.*

Mukhtyar C. et al. 2009. "EULAR recommendations for the management of primary small and medium vessel vasculitis." *Ann Rheum Dis.*

Ode, Kazu, et al. 2014. "High-dose intravenous immunoglobulin therapy induces and maintains complete remission for polyarteritis nodosa." *Case Reports in Internal Medicine.*

Ostojic, Predrag and Ivan R Jeremic. 2017. "Managing refractory cryoglobulinemic vasculitis: challenges and solutions." *Journal of Inflammation Research.*

Piazza, Gregory and Mark A. Creager. 2010. "Thrombangiitis Obliterans." *Circulation.*

Rife, Eileen and Abraham Gedalia. 2020. "Kawasaki Disease: an Update." *Current Rheumatology Reports.*

Ritter, James M. and others. *A Textbook of Clinical Pharmacology and Therapeutics: Fifth Edition.*

Roaa S. Alsolaimani, et al. 2016 " Severe Intracranial Involvement in Giant Cell Arteritis: 5 Cases and Literature Review " *The Journal of Rheumatology.*

Russell, James P. and Lawrence E. Gibson. 2006. "Primary cutaneous small vessel vasculitis: approach to diagnosis and treatment." *International Journal of Dermatology.*

Sarah L. et al. 2020. "British Society for Rheumatology guidelines on diagnosis and treatment of giant cell arteritis."

Teixeira V. et al. 2019. "Efficacy and safety of rituximab in the treatment of eosinophilic granulomatosis with polyangiitis." *RMD Open.*

Terrier, Benjamin and Patrice Cacoub. 2013. "Cryoglobulinemic vasculitis: an update." *Curr Opin Rheumatol.*

Vallianou K. et al. 2020. "A case report of hypocomplementemic urticarial vasculitis presenting with membranoproliferative glomerulonephritis." *BMC Nephrology.*

Vijayakumar A. et al. 2013. "Thrombangiitis Obliterans (Buerger's Disease)-Current Practices." *International Journal of Inflammation.*

Wallace, Zachary S. and Eli M. Miloslavsky. 2020. "Management of ANCA associated vasculitis." *BMJ.*

West, Dr. Sterling and Dr. Jason Kolfenbach. Rheumatology Secrets Book, Fourth Edition.

Yates M. et al. 2016. "EULAR/ERA-EDTA recommendations for management of ANCA-associated vasculitis." *Ann Rheum Dis.*

Zanatta, Elisabetta, et al. 2019. "The role of plasma exchange in the management of autoimmune disorders." *British Journal of Hematology.*

Zarka F. et al. "A Review of Primary Vasculitis Mimickers Based on Chapel Hill Consensus Classification." *International Journal of Rheumatology.*

www.ingramcontent.com/pod-product-compliance
Lightning Source LLC
Chambersburg PA
CBHW070636220526
45466CB00001B/188